I AM JUST A WOMAN (SECOND EDITION)

MY STORY OF DOMESTIC VIOLENCE, RECOVERY FROM PTSD & WAKING UP TO A WHOLE NEW LIFE

MARY SCHILLER

a.k.a.
LUCY JOHNSON

WWW.MARYSCHILLER.COM

Copyright © 2017 by Mary Schiller

All rights reserved.

No part of this book may be reproduced in any form or by any electronic or mechanical means, including information storage and retrieval systems, without written permission from the author, except for the use of brief quotations in a book review.

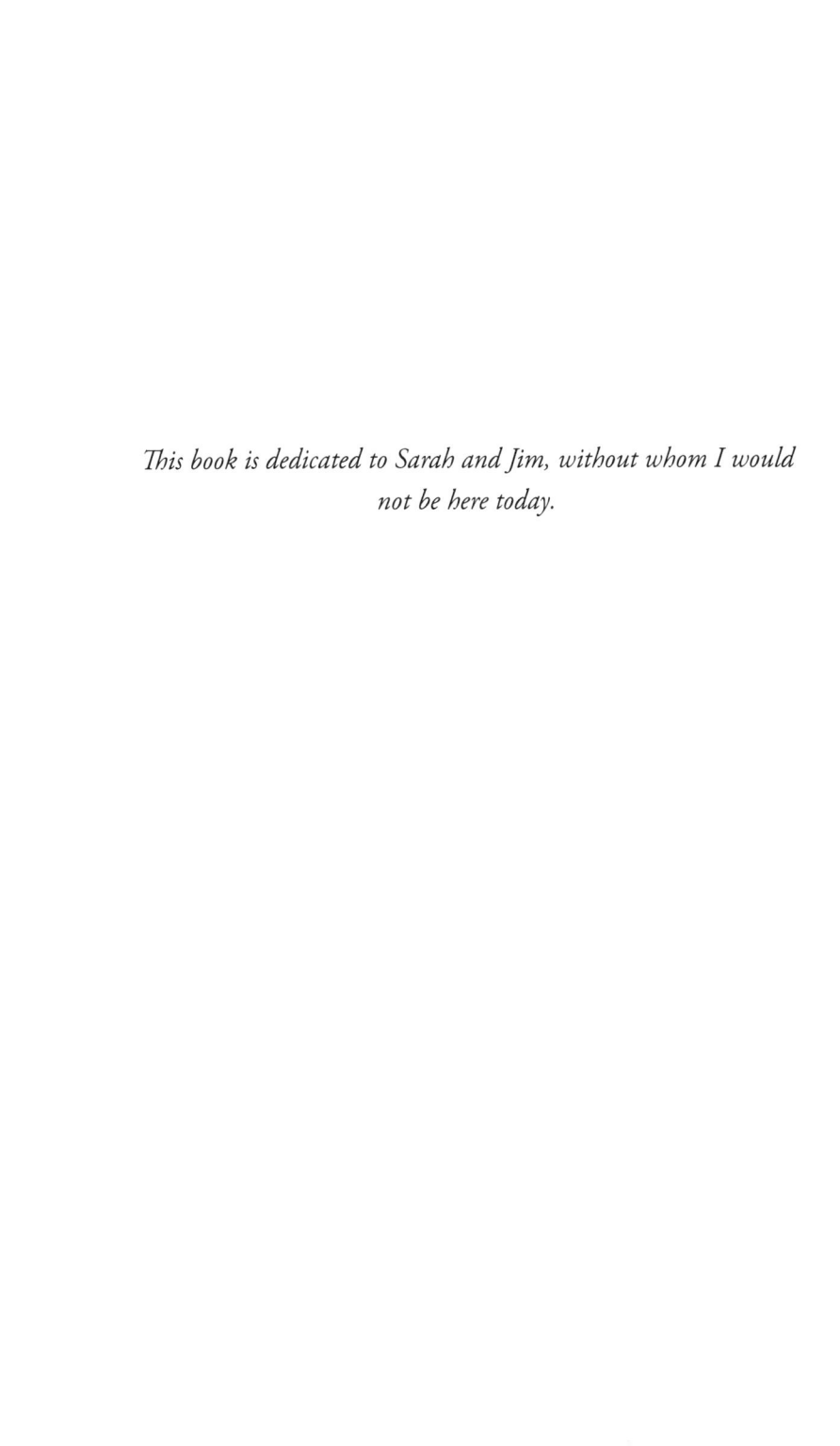

This book is dedicated to Sarah and Jim, without whom I would not be here today.

CONTENTS

Prologue … 1

Introduction … 5

PART I
1. 1983 Was the Year I Got Married … 9
2. A Young Woman Meets a Young Man … 11
3. The Word "Just" … 15
4. Postcards from the Edge … 17
5. Did it Really Happen? … 19
6. Yes, It Was … 21
7. Stress, Over the Long Haul … 23
8. Race … 25
9. You Never Know What You've Got 'Till it's Gone … 29

PART II
10. 3 A.M. … 35
11. 4 A.M. … 39
12. Fact vs. Truth … 41
13. In the Body … 43
14. Parental Consent … 47
15. First Sign of Trouble … 49
16. Back from the Honeymoon … 51
17. Counselor No. 1 … 55
18. No Drinking, No Drugs … 57
19. Counselor No. 2 … 59
20. Walking on Broken Glass … 61
21. I Know What the Questions Are … 63
22. Mind Games … 65

23. Broken Memories 67
24. Screaming 69
25. Last Glimpse of Julian 71
26. Never 75
27. Wanting a Baby 77
28. "Another Bitch" 81
29. Two Whole Weeks 83
30. In the Present Tense 85
31. The Deepest Grief 87
32. Blurting It Out 91
33. A Jab in the Back Can Be a Good Thing 95
34. A Witness 99
35. Miscarriage 103
36. Dinner Plate 107
37. Sad Mother-In-Law 111
38. Crossing Over 115
39. Turning Points 117
40. Newspaper 119
41. K-Y 121
42. Feeling Ugly 123
43. In Between 125
44. On the Sofa 127
45. Existence 131
46. Mexican Vacation 133
47. Who to Turn To 135
48. Suitcase 139
49. Mental List 141
50. Fear of Dying 145
51. The Night Before 147
52. It Was a Sunny Day 149

PART III
53. I Thought It Was Over 155
54. Embarrassment 157
55. Immediate Aftermath 161

56. Who Is She?	163
57. A Photo of the Real Me	165
58. Credit Card Lesson	167
59. Solicitation	169
60. Domestic Violence Therapist	171
61. Flinching	175
62. Confusion	177
63. Tranquilizer	181
64. $900	183
65. Record of Lies, Destroyed	187
66. Blessing	191
67. Lost in My 20s … and My 30s and 40s	193
68. Jacket	195
69. Child Psychologist	199

PART IV

70. The Light was Pink	205
71. Mandated Reporter	209
72. The Authorities	211
73. Children's Hospital	215
74. Running	219
75. My Mother	221
76. More Authorities	225
77. Flowers and Screens	227
78. The Question	229
79. Reprimand	231
80. Canada or Mexico	235
81. Court-Appointed Psychiatrist	237
82. Depositions and Court Appearances	241
83. The Ruling	243
84. What Now?	247
85. Lydia	251
86. Naive, but Vigilant	253
87. Easter 1992	255
88. LA Riots, Major Decision	257

89. Where to Go	261
90. No Help for Sarah	263
91. Talking to Mark	265
92. The Arrangement	267
93. The Body	271
94. Trauma's Health Effects	277
95. "You Blame Me"	279
96. Her Screams	281
97. Fatigue	285
98. Rape / Forgiveness	287
99. Halfway / Headaches	291
100. So Many Birthdays	293

PART V

101. Never-Ending Nightmare	297
102. Molestation = Many Forms	301
103. Jim	305
104. Sam	307
105. Closer to the Truth	309
106. Meeting	311
107. Loss	315
108. Ex Parte	317
109. Bedtime	319
110. Letter to Mark	323
111. Sarah's Disclosure, and Mine	325
112. All Over Again	327
113. Police	329
114. Dr. Chen	331
115. Shocking Information about Mark	333
116. A Day in Court, Part 1	337
117. A Day in Court, Part 2	339
118. Bill, the Counselor	345
119. Trying to be Normal	347
120. "Nothing."	349
121. Help for Sarah	353

122. A Deposition	355
123. Interminable	357
124. Still Controlling?	361
125. All of us Together	363
126. Cards & Grandmother	365
127. Normal?	367
Epilogue	371
1. The Happy Ending Starts Here	373
2. A Chance Encounter with a Book	379
3. The Truth	383
4. A Turning Point	389
5. Motherhood, Reborn	393
6. The Happy Ending Continues	397
7. What to Do Next	401
About the Author	403
Also by Mary Schiller	405

PROLOGUE

When I originally wrote and self published *I Am Just A Woman* in 2012, I used the pseudonym of Lucy Johnson. Why? It's pretty simple: I was afraid to put this book out into the world with my real name on it, for a whole host of reasons.

It was the right decision back then.

Today, I'm making a different decision: to publish a new edition of the book using my real name (with the consent of my current husband and daughter); and, even more importantly, to include an epilogue that describes the miraculous changes that have occurred in my life since 2014. (Note that everyone else's names remain pseudonyms.)

THE INTRODUCTION AND FIVE PARTS OF THE BOOK ARE JUST AS THEY WERE IN 2012.

I have left the book as-is because of the beautiful feedback I have received over the years from people who have been encouraged by reading my story. Yes, I could make some edits and changes to it, but I have chosen to leave it alone and let it stand on its own two feet (kind of like me).

WHAT'S NEW IS THE EPILOGUE.

If you don't typically read epilogues in books, I urge you to read this one. In it, I explain what I discovered in 2014 that not only dissolved all my symptoms of post-traumatic stress disorder (PTSD) nearly overnight, but also completely changed my life for the better.

Never in my wildest dreams did I think I could live the way I do now: carefree, and without chronic stress, worry or fear.

In short, I am a new person. Or rather, I'm the person I always was, and so much more.

The best news is, there is nothing special about me. What helped me can help anyone and everyone.

If you're reading this book because you have been touched in some way by domestic violence and/or want relief from trauma (or know someone who fits that description), then please read the epilogue when you get there. I wrote it especially for you.

And if you're reading this book because you simply want

to improve your life — you want to live with less fear and anxiety, and with more happiness and freedom — the epilogue is also for you.

THERE IS HOPE. MORE THAN YOU CAN IMAGINE.

Now begins the original *I Am Just A Woman* …
　　Much love to you,
　　Mary, a.k.a. Lucy

INTRODUCTION

I am just a woman.

There is nothing particularly special about me. I'm not rich or famous. I haven't had a brilliant career. I haven't made a name for myself in any way.

The words people use to describe me are "brave" and "strong." Over the past few years, as I have come to understand my life's experiences, I have learned to hold on to those words. They are meaningful to me. If I had the choice between being "rich and famous" or "brave and strong," I would choose the latter.

But in the end, I am just a woman.

I know other people have life-changing experiences every day. We read their stories in the paper and online, and we see them on TV.

My story hasn't appeared on TV or in the newspaper. And I haven't spoken about my life with many people. But the experiences I chronicle here not only changed my life, they changed me.

I'm sure some will wonder why I've chosen to publish this book under a pseudonym – Lucy Johnson is not my real name. Considering the rash of memoirs in recent years that have turned out to be fraudulent, some may even wonder if I'm a real person, or if my story is real.

I am, and it is. People who know my life will probably recognize me. But otherwise, no one will know. I've never been an attention seeker. Wallflower … that's what I've been, and how I've felt, most of my life.

I've changed the real names of everyone because I am writing about their lives, too. And while everything I've written is true, it does involve other people. Sure, autobiographies generally use people's real names. For me, it just doesn't feel comfortable.

Ironically, I have felt invisible inside my own life for many years, so being anonymous inside a pseudonym feels rather normal to me.

I have just one hope for this book: that it can help another person out there, a woman who is, or has been, in the situation in which I found myself back in 1983.

PART I

1983 WAS THE YEAR I GOT MARRIED

The year 1983 was the most pivotal year of my life – actually beginning the fall of 1982.

I was a senior in college, feeling burned out by school. I was in a major that wasn't quite suited to me, but I had found a niche within it where I excelled. Even though I was tired of being a student, I considered the possibility of continuing to graduate school right after finishing my bachelor's.

In the fall of 1982, I spoke to a couple of professors in the field I was considering. They were encouraging, because they knew my skills and aptitude in the area of study (music history). But they also said that I needed to be certain of what I wanted from my PhD. If I wasn't totally committed, I should wait a year and see how I felt at that point.

When I look back on this period, I realize that those conversations were very influential on some of the decisions I made. In fact, I wasn't completely certain I wanted the life of a college professor. While I knew I could handle the academics, I wasn't ready to commit.

If only I had.

Instead, I got married – a decision I would never have made if I had only been … well, older and wiser.

But I was young and, frankly, naive. I didn't know much about the psychological challenges I was being confronted with — in the people in my life at the time, not me — and I couldn't have named them back then: among them, depression, suicidal thoughts, sociopath-type behavior, psychosis. I type those words now, and they truly are terrifying.

I didn't know what the word "terrifying" meant back then. I do now.

A YOUNG WOMAN MEETS A YOUNG MAN

I loved my days as an undergraduate student at UCLA. The campus was gorgeous, all flowering trees and grassy lawns, with the feel of an Ivy League (without the price tag). Even at the time, I remember thinking how lucky I was to spend my days in such a beautiful place. I made friends and had fun. I worked hard and struggled in some of my classes (like macro economics – what was I thinking taking that class?). Overall, it was a joyous time.

When I was a freshman, I met a young man named Julian. He was the best friend of one of my closest friends during college, Scott. Scott and Julian had gone to high school together, they still played in a band together, and they were two of the nicest guys you could ever hope to meet. If you were the mother of a college-aged daughter, you couldn't have asked for a more honorable pair of ... yes, gentlemen for your daughter to have as protectors/friends.

Scott and I were just friends, good friends. No "funny

business" between us. He often asked my opinion on what he should wear on a date, because he was nearly completely color blind – purple was a total mystery to him, which I always thought was rather sad. Can you imagine never seeing the deep, rich color of an eggplant? His favorite question to ask me was, "Does this go together? What does that even mean, 'go together?' Makes no sense to me!" Occasionally our friends and I would dress him up in something ridiculous, but tempting as it was because Scott was so good natured, we'd never let him out the door like that.

Scott was genuine and kind, with a huge heart (and a typically '80s hairstyle to match). He listened to me when I was down, and he celebrated with me when I was up. I hope I did the same for him during those years at UCLA.

Toward the end of our freshman year, he asked if I wanted to come along with him to see his younger friend Julian in Julian's senior high school musical, "Oklahoma!" I thought it would be a lot of fun, so I went along. Their high school was nearby, in Pasadena, and all of their friends would be there, some of whom I already had met at UCLA and liked very much.

My first glimpse of Julian wasn't a glimpse at all. It was his voice, singing in a deep baritone from offstage: "There's a bright golden haze on the meadow … ."

As soon as I saw him onstage, I was immediately taken with him. Not love at first sight — I don't believe in that — but certainly I was intrigued. He was tall, with honey-colored skin (what he later would describe to me as "coffee with cream"), and he had such presence. I couldn't take my eyes off of him.

After the play, Scott and I went backstage to congratulate Julian on his performance, which was magnificent (speaking purely objectively, of course). Julian was there with his girlfriend — about as opposite from me as possible, petite and cute — and I felt my stomach drop a little. He shook my hand and thanked me for coming to the play. And Scott and I drove back to the dorm to finish out our freshman year uneventfully.

Not quite. Julian and I saw each other one more time before my freshman year at college ended.

It was the last day of the school year, and Scott and I decided we'd spend it together. We had grown very close — again, just as friends — and we had a lot of fun hanging out. He played the guitar and sang, and he wrote songs, and we'd have a great time making up goofy lyrics about our professors and classmates and living in the dorms.

We hadn't yet seen the "Star Wars" sequel, "The Empire Strikes Back," so we thought that going to the movie would be a nice way to end our freshman year. Plus, it was unbearably hot that June of 1980, and the cool air conditioning of a movie theater was just too hard to resist.

At the last minute, Scott's friend Julian called and said he was coming into the city. Scott asked me if it would be all right if Julian joined us.

"Would it be all right?" I said to myself, my heart jumping more than a little. "Of course, that would be great," I replied, in my calmest voice.

Julian picked us up at our dorm, and we drove to the

theater in his gold Mustang. Once we were inside, these two young gentlemen — really, they were true gentlemen — asked where I'd like to sit. I chose to sit between them.

As the lights went down, I experienced a moment in time I will never forget. I felt such a zing, a literal zing, just being near Julian. Without saying a word to each other to that effect, I knew Julian felt the same. Isn't that strange, how people can literally have "chemistry"?

Writing about it this way seems a bit self indulgent, and even a little corny and sentimental. But as you get older, you look back on moments that were special to you. And you revel in them just a little: you put yourself back into that theater seat, with the lights dimming and the music rising, and your heart beating a little faster because you're sitting within an inch or two of someone you find attractive.

This was the closest I had yet been to Julian, and it was truly electric.

We went our separate ways after the movie, and my heart broke a little, knowing I was going back home for the summer and wouldn't see him — maybe ever, since I thought he still had a girlfriend. I didn't realize how magical a summer it would be.

THE WORD "JUST"

I inherited the word "just" from my mother, who probably inherited it from her mother. It's one of those qualifier words that take away the power from a statement.

I am a woman.

I am just a woman.

My mother was a person of little self-esteem, the youngest child in a somewhat difficult family — although I wouldn't know the details, personally. All of my grandparents died long before I was born, and I never knew my extended family at all. My beautiful mother died a long time ago, so she isn't here to answer any more of my questions.

I worded the title of this book intentionally with the word "just," because for me, it represents this feeling of essential inadequacy that has permeated most of my life. Even now, at mid life, I have not outgrown the "just." The experiences I'm writing about here, in fact, reinforced this feeling of inadequacy that I am now working to overcome

The book title also makes me think of all the times my mother couched her opinions behind an uneasy smile and laugh, as if she didn't really know enough about the topic — whatever it was — to offer an opinion that mattered.

Of course, that wasn't true. She was a woman of deep understanding of human nature, always able to read people in a way that was, truly, amazing. She had a gift for seeing beyond any mask or front that a person wore, and, I have to say, she was right nearly 100 percent of the time.

I should have listened to her more often, especially concerning the man I married in 1983.

But in 1980, when I had met and started to fall in love with Julian, my mother sensed what was going on between us. I thought she did not approve of this potential love affair, as she tried — in vain, ultimately to convince me not to start dating Julian.

Not having her sense of how to read people, I realize now that I was completely wrong about how she felt. She may have had a few misgivings, but now I understand that she was trying to protect me from my father, who would never approve my relationship with Julian.

Why? Because Julian is "coffee with cream," the product of a white father from Spain and an African-American mother from the Midwest, and I am solely "cream," of Swedish ancestry. The color of one's skin matters to a lot of people.

That's something I "just" didn't understand as I ventured into that lovely summer and fall of 1980.

POSTCARDS FROM THE EDGE

※

*R*ight before you fall in love, there's that glorious tipsy feeling, as if you're literally standing on a precipice with your toes slipping over the edge. Your head spins, your heart pounds, and then you lose your balance and take the plunge.

The summer of 1980 was an edgy, tingly time. I felt alive and pretty and all those wonderful feelings. I spent the summer at my parents' home, and Julian was abroad on a trip to Europe — his first as a young adult — to spend time with his father's family in Spain and travel to different European capitals. He had since ended his relationship with the girl I met backstage at his senior high school play and, as I soon discovered, he cared for me a great deal.

At each place he visited, he would buy a postcard, write something lovely, and send it to me.

Pretty soon, my mailbox and my heart were filled with the words on these cards. If only I had saved them! I would love to be able to read them again. Being courted from afar like this was so romantic, especially because in those days, it wasn't instant communication: no email or text messages. I held each card in my hands and had time to read it over and over again, savoring the words. Like when Julian visited Paris, and wrote something like, "This city is meant for lovers."

I knew he was picturing us there together, standing on a bridge overlooking the Seine, taking in the Paris landscape basked in golden light.

Later, Julian told me that before he had even sent the first postcard, he had asked Scott's permission to take me out on a date, just to make sure Scott didn't have romantic feelings toward me. When Scott expressed his enthusiasm for the idea, Julian felt free to express himself on all those beautiful cards.

When he returned to the States to attend Cal State Northridge and I started my sophomore year UCLA in the fall, Julian and I started dating officially. He chose to live with Scott and three other roommates in an apartment nearer UCLA than Northridge, so it would be easier for us to spend time together.

Despite the reservations expressed to me by my mother and even a couple of my friends, I saw no reason why I shouldn't date Julian. I still, to this day, don't understand the point of view that says dating someone of another race is wrong.

As time went on, though, I wasn't strong enough to withstand the pressure. And Julian had some difficulties ahead, as well.

DID IT REALLY HAPPEN?

*S*ometimes things happen to you that, even at the time, you wonder if they are actually real. Even now, 28 years after it happened, I still ask myself if it really, truly did.

But I know the answer. All these hours, days, months, years, decades later, it's still difficult for me to think about the event that occurred in the early morning hours of Oct. 23, 1983.

Because you just don't expect the man you married just hours earlier to rape you.

That's a tough sentence to think, let alone type and see in print. And the thing is, few people believe it's possible. After all, how could you be raped by your husband on your wedding night? Doesn't that go against everything we've come to believe about what's supposed to happen on a wedding night?

The answer is, yes, it goes against everything we believe. And yes, it did really happen. That moment changed my life.

Changed *me*.

I am not, nor will I ever be — as much as I've tried to fight it — the person I was before I was raped by my husband. That woman is gone and will never come back.

All these years later, I am working to accept the new person who lives inside me. She seems like a foreigner much of the time. Every day since Oct. 23, 1983, I've looked in the mirror and not recognized the person staring back at me. Her eyes have a blue, icy emptiness. Now that the lines are creeping in, she looks even sadder to me, despite the dimples that still show when she smiles.

I keep wondering if, one day, I will become whole again. I've worked and continue to work on repairing what I can and trying to accept the rest. Maybe this is the best I can do. Maybe I need to stop chastising myself for not being more … whatever it is. More me?

I'm not there yet. And the memory of that early morning event is still with me in the most starkly realistic way a memory can present itself in the mind and body.

YES, IT WAS

❦

When I think back on some of the happiest times of my life — there have been some happy times, thankfully — I remember the autumn of 1980 as one of them. Julian and I had fallen in love, and we created some beautiful memories.

Like driving in his new white Mustang — the gold one bit the dust — west on Sunset Boulevard to the beach, with the top down, listening to Steely Dan and breathing in the slightly salty, slightly smoggy, air. Or going to the movies in Westwood, or heading to the clubs for band gigs — for his and Scott's band and others. (I was always amazed that we never got carded in these nightclubs. Surely we didn't look old enough to drink, did we?)

I spent time with Julian's parents, and his circle of friends became my circle of friends. Of course, we already had Scott in common, but through the two of them I met some of the most wonderful people. We'd watch MTV (new at the time!), play music, sing, play board games ... oh, and we'd study sometimes, too.

While all of those activities were great fun, what I remember most is the way I felt. I am so fortunate to have experienced the deep, intense love that comes when one is young. It didn't matter how many times I saw Julian, my body still felt that electric zing every single time he entered the room. When he smiled at me, said my name, and — how's this for romantic? — when he wrote and sang songs just for me, I felt my whole being just melt into an easy peace.

Today, we don't live near each other and we have our own lives. I don't see Julian anymore; we haven't spoken for a while. But he asked me one time, several years ago, if I agreed with him that even though it was young love, it was love, not infatuation. "Was it real?" he asked me. "Because it felt real to me."

Yes, I said. *It was real.*

And it was wonderful.

STRESS, OVER THE LONG HAUL

⚭

*R*ecently, I watched a National Geographic documentary about stress. Of course, we all know that stress affects us in myriad ways: some good, most not.

I think about the chronic stress I experienced, starting Oct. 23, 1983, and ending — mostly — in April of 2001. The level of stress is hard to describe in words. I remember feeling as though my insides were twisted like bent metal, my back was somehow broken in a million places and wouldn't hold me up, and as if I were facing a loaded gun, 24 hours a day.

The worst part is, I could do absolutely nothing about the situation. Over the years, I have taunted myself with the notion that I could have. But that's just not the reality.

I did not know the term "domestic violence" until I had already walked — more like run — away from my home. A couple of weeks later, I found myself sitting in a musty, beige office at the LA courthouse waiting for a mandatory counseling session to begin. Mandatory, because if you had children and were getting divorced, the court believed it best for you to talk to one of their counselors.

The words were written on a poster on the wall: "The Cycle of Domestic Violence." It had a checklist of about a dozen ways that a spouse abuses the other: "If you have experienced even one of these, then you are a victim of domestic violence."

I had checked all of them.

Looking back on that day, at the time I thought the worst was over. I thought, OK, now I know what this is called, this "thing" I've been trying to deal with since 1983. I can start to work on it.

But my stress level was only going to get more intense following my marital escape in 1990. I did not know that a new kind of horror would continue for 11 more years. I can only guess what the stress did to my body. In many ways, I feel grateful that, somehow, I've managed not to show it too much on the outside.

If I'm honest with myself, I know that I haven't let go of it completely, either. The stress from those years still lives inside me, because it has changed who I am.

I may be strong. And I may even be brave. But I'm not sure who I am.

RACE

Julian and I dated throughout most of my college career, starting in the fall of my sophomore year through March of my senior year at UCLA.

We still felt all that same electricity between us, but the relationship began unraveling about mid-way through. There were two major reasons for our troubles, the first of which may seem obvious: we were of different races, and my parents did not approve.

They absolutely loved Julian — as a friend for me. He was polite, well spoken, educated, smart, and truly talented. He was definitely going to make something of himself, as he had (still does have!) a knack for sales like nobody's business. My parents could tell that he would be successful one day.

But not with their (white) daughter standing beside him.

Secretly, I think my parents wished I would date Scott, instead: the young man who was my friend, and one of Julian's best friends. But Scott and I would never be more than friends.

Julian's parents were lovely people who always welcomed me with open arms whenever I visited their home in Pasadena. Julian's father was an excellent cook; my mother even joined all of us for dinner one evening at Julian's parents' home. She raved about the meal — lamb, potatoes, and the most amazing paella ever—for months afterward.

The pressure of my parents' disapproval weighed heavily on Julian and me, so much so that after about a year of dating him, I lied and told my parents we had broken up — which we hadn't. Understandably, Julian began to feel like I was ashamed of him. Of course I wasn't. I loved Julian. But to enforce their point, my parents had threatened to stop paying for my education if I kept seeing him. One time, on a visit home, my father started putting my belongings outside the front door and said I was no longer his daughter if I continued my relationship with Julian.

My mother was more understanding of our situation, but I think she feared the rift that was being created between my father and me. My father never yelled, ever, but as the episode with my belongings may suggest, he let his displeasure be known in other ways. In the end, lying to my parents seemed like the only choice.

Race simply was not, and is not, a problem for me when it comes to dating or marriage. To this day, I have trouble understanding my parents' perspective. If you changed his skin to white, he would have been the "perfect" guy, in their eyes.

It made me sad, really. And I think this situation

contributed to the other problem Julian developed while in school: depression.

I remember being in my apartment my senior year of college, with Julian in the living room listening to music, I think it was The Police — on a turntable, back in those days. I went into the bedroom for a moment to get something, not sure what. When I came out into the living room, Julian was gone.

By this point, more than two years after we started dating, I had experienced Julian's moodiness. That's what I called it, at least: moodiness. I didn't really understand what was going on with him. He would get so down, there were times when he literally wouldn't leave his room. At all. For days.

Then other times, he would be more like himself, upbeat and creative, energetic and funny.

I don't know if it was some sort of bi-polar condition or what; all I knew back then was that he was "moody." It was stressful to watch him go through these tough times without being able to do anything to help him.

His ups and downs may have been related to our relationship, the fact that I had to hide us being together from my parents and family. They simply could not accept the fact that he was black, and I was white. Looking back on it now, I'm sure there were other reasons for Julian's apparent depression, perhaps college pressure or even biochemical changes over which he had no control.

That particular evening, with the music playing on the turntable, I felt a sense of panic overtake me. I had a flash of another moment with Julian, where I was driving on the 405 freeway with him in the passenger seat. Suddenly, he opened the passenger door and threatened to jump. With all my strength, I held onto the wheel with my left hand, reached all the way over to the door with my right, and slammed it shut.

In my empty living room that night, I quickly thought of places he might have gone. I immediately ran out onto the terrace — I lived on the 15th floor — and looked over the edge. Thank God, nothing.

I then took the elevator down to the garage, to the area where Julian normally parked his car. His white Mustang was still there, but no Julian.

Then, with my heart really racing, I shot up in the elevator to the roof, where there was a tennis court. To my shock, there he was, standing near the edge and looking as if he might do the unthinkable.

I wish I could remember what I said to calm him down. I'm sure adrenaline is what has erased that conversation from my memory. All I know for certain is that he didn't jump. At that very moment, much as I loved him, I realized the stress of this situation – this moodiness – was too difficult for me to bear.

YOU NEVER KNOW WHAT YOU'VE GOT 'TILL IT'S GONE

Breaking up with someone has to be one of the worst things you can do. It hurts you, it hurts the other person, and it just hurts, period.

I met Julian in a park. It wasn't a very pretty park, in the center of the San Fernando Valley. There were some ducks and geese there that looked like they'd seen better days, with their matted and dirty feathers. The grass was mostly brown dirt, even though it was springtime, 1983. But we put a blanket on the ground and talked for a while, and I tried to steel myself for what I had to say to him.

"I've started seeing someone else," I blurted out.

He sat in silence. I don't think he believed me. But it was true.

I had met Mark a couple of weeks earlier, on a blind date. I was doing an internship at a record company and, through Mark's sister Lynn who worked there, had been set up on the date. The first date itself was rather funny, because, no kidding, Mark lost his wallet and I ended up having to pay. Mark was positively mortified, assuming I thought he was lying. But he was so upset about it, I knew he was telling the truth. His apologies were endearing, and we had a nice evening. I had seen him several times in the past couple of weeks, and I knew in my heart that I couldn't see Julian anymore.

At that moment, telling Julian about Mark, I didn't know how serious my relationship with Mark would become, and how quickly. But I knew that I couldn't hurt Julian by seeing Mark at the same time and lying about it.

After he accepted what I had told him, Julian asked if we could kiss one last time. We did, and surprisingly, I didn't feel any of that old electricity. I felt deeply sad about that, because I still loved Julian, but I could not invest any more of myself in our relationship. The difficulties with my family, his apparent depression (although remember, I called it "moodiness"), the ups and downs of everything were just too much for me.

At the time, Mark seemed like a safe harbor. He had already graduated from college and was developing a business, one in which he excelled. He was smart, charming and funny. I was becoming friendly with his three older sisters, and his parents seemed decent, upon first meeting.

Mark also was a rebound, though I was too immature to recognize it at the time.

Was it all a mistake? It's hard to answer that. On the surface, it would seem that it was, ending my relationship with

Julian and taking up with Mark so fast. The choice I made cost me dearly, and caused other people to suffer, too.

But how can we look back at ourselves, our 22-year-old selves, and make that kind of a judgment? Is there a way to forgive ourselves for making a young person's mistake that affects the rest of our lives?

PART II

3 A.M.

Our wedding was Oct. 22, 1983 — a Saturday. Mark and I scheduled it late in the evening so that Mark's relatives could attend, because many of them were orthodox Jewish.

Even with that plan, the wedding started much later than expected because of a massive accident on the freeway, just before the exit people had to take to get to the church. Yes, we were married in a church, despite his Jewish background. It was important to me, and not being religious, Mark agreed to it.

So the wedding ceremony didn't start until about 8:30 p.m.

After the ceremony came the photos, which took forever because the photographer was not only slow, but overly meticulous and incredibly annoying. Then on to the reception, which, thankfully, was a lot of fun. My friends were musicians – Scott, who sang during the ceremony, and several others — took over from the band, at one point, and played a couple of special songs for us. People danced until all hours. We had a wonderful time. Even years later, people who attended our reception said it was the best wedding reception they'd been to.

After all the festivities, Mark and I left under a shower of rice and headed for a hotel near LAX, because our plane for Mexico was leaving very early the next morning. By the time we got to the hotel, well after 1 a.m., I was tired and starving. Typical bride: I hadn't eaten much at all before, during or after the wedding. So Mark went downstairs (room service was finished for the night) and brought back a salad for me; food service was closed, and a salad was the best he could do. It tasted great to me.

By the time I finished eating and we had talked about our big day, it was nearly 3 a.m., and I was dead tired. We had to be at the airport by 7 a.m., and all I wanted was a couple of hours of sleep. I couldn't remember ever feeling so exhausted.

Mark, however, had other things on his mind. For me, I didn't see any big deal about actually "consummating" the marriage at that very moment. After all, we had been sleeping together for months, so that was nothing new. And in truth, I wanted to save that moment for our beautiful honeymoon spot in Mexico. I thought it would be more romantic that way.

My gentle, "Let's get some sleep and celebrate in Mexico" was quickly rebuffed with a loud, "I'm not waiting until then."

In an instant, it was like he flipped a switch, and suddenly he wasn't Mark anymore. His words — spoken forcefully, in a tone I had heard only once before, and not directed at me — were accompanied by glaring eyes and clenched teeth.

He grabbed me so hard around my arm, that I could feel the bruise forming right away. Because he did manual labor for a living, he was incredibly strong. It only took him seconds to overpower me.

There I was, still wearing my leaving-the-reception dress of white with black polka dots, being raped by my new husband inside a hotel near LAX.

While he did it, he said nothing, and I said nothing. I just felt the weight of his body on top of me and his hands holding me not with love, but with hate, and I tried not to look into the eyes that I no longer recognized.

4 A.M.

After my husband of just a few hours forcibly raped me on our wedding night, a strange thing happened.

My mind literally went blank. It was like my body was moving — I got up from the bed, took off my now slightly ripped reception dress, changed into something else and brushed my teeth — without feeling the slightest connection to my mind.

A sense of total blankness.

And if I'm honest, I have to say that it persists in some lesser form today, 28 years later.

At that moment on Oct. 23, 1983, I lost my *self*. My judgment, my self-esteem, my faith — everything vanished.

At 4 a.m., I wasn't the same person I had been at 3 a.m. I don't know where she went, but she disappeared and has never been seen or heard from since.

If my husband hadn't become violent and abusive with me in the days, months and years after the rape, things might have been different. But the rape was only the first of many violent incidents to come, including more rape and other things that I could never have foreseen.

But all I knew at 4 a.m. was that I was a blank. Now, of course, I realize that I went into shock.

Someone reading this may be thinking, "Why didn't you just gather your things right then and there, and walk out the door?"

To that, I would say: "Have you ever seen a trauma or crime victim, who is in shock, do something 'normal'?" People in this state of mind are not thinking clearly. They're injured, physically and mentally, and often go into denial about their experience. I didn't even want to acknowledge what happened to me. I kept asking myself, over and over again, Did it really happen?

Before I had time to think or take action or make sense of anything, it was time to go to the airport and get on our honeymoon flight to Mexico.

I started my married life, at age 22, as a traumatized rape victim.

FACT VS. TRUTH

Even though they're painful to write about, in the scheme of things, facts are relatively easy. I can recount incidents that occurred, and I can delineate the facts and let them speak for themselves.

As real as the facts may be, they don't tell the whole story. The whole story rests inside the human being who has had the experience. It's the experience itself, both in body and mind, that forms the truth. And truth is different from fact.

So what is the truth of 3 a.m., Oct. 23, 1983, and the events that came after it? Well, I've written a bit about the blankness I felt, and still feel to a certain extent. But I haven't written about what eventually colored that blankness.

First was the shock. After the initial shock wore off, a strange and baffling form of denial set in.

I became a woman obsessed with trying to sort it out: what happened really didn't happen, because it simply couldn't have happened. And then I'd say to myself, But it did happen.

Then I'd question myself: Didn't it? Imagine a clock with a pendulum swinging from side to side. That's how my mind felt: for hours, then days, then weeks, months and years after that initial rape on my wedding night. Did it happen? No. Did it happen? Yes. Did it happen? No. Did it happen? Yes.

Over the years, "it" began to refer to lots of actions by Mark against me: raping, cursing, throwing things, screaming, threatening with death, choking, grabbing, shoving, knocking down, berating, name calling, playing endless mind games, cheating with other women.

And always … the pendulum, swinging back and forth in my mind. No. But yes. *No!* But yes. *NO!*

Some things are just too difficult for the mind to bear. Even when the body is experiencing the physical truth of all of it, the mind continues to deny. I've come to believe it's a form of self-protection, and in the case of domestic violence, "protection" is literal.

In that denial lies the truth. But sometimes, it can take years to really allow yourself to accept the truth and wake up from the trauma you're experiencing. That's what happened to me.

IN THE BODY

I read a quote recently by Allen Ginsberg, something along the lines of, "Writing is in the body." This statement reflects my experience of writing this book. It has brought up bodily feelings — tightness in my chest, shortness of breath, sweating — that demonstrate the truth of our memories being held in the body.

After the initial rape, my body went through a lot of trauma. I can recall feeling as though my ears were ringing constantly, a humming that I could never mute. To this day, that ringing has not gone away. On our honeymoon in Mexico, I had stomach problems that were not caused by drinking the water or eating the food. I was nauseated and had no appetite. I was also stung by some sort of insect, on my cheek, and my face swelled for a couple of days.

And of course, Mark wanted to have sex while we were there. It's difficult to describe what went through my mind and body during those times. I remember my body rebelling against the act itself, so that the sex became quite painful for me. This had never happened to me before. I wasn't present, in any sense of the word. If I had to draw an analogy, I would describe myself as a literal wooden board whenever I engaged in sex with Mark.

He didn't care.

Before he raped me, our sex life had been pretty good. I enjoyed it.

Afterward, I was a wooden board. But … he didn't care. He did what he wanted to do, and that was it. There was no apology, no concern expressed for me, nothing.

My body was telling me, of course, that this man wasn't safe for me to be with. But that pendulum in my mind kept swinging back and forth between the truth and the denial of it.

There also was a strong element of fear that kept me there, during the honeymoon and beyond. Suddenly I was afraid of Mark, and even though I didn't articulate it, I knew he was capable of much more violence. My days and nights became consumed by the idea of self-preservation.

It's hard not to feel saddened by the tremendous loss I experienced. My 22-year-old body — I must say, it was a nice one — was basically left for dead for many years. Today, I am still grieving for my physical self. We only have one chance to be that age, in our physical prime, ready for all the joy and excitement life offers. That joy was taken away from me, by someone I thought I knew, someone I thought loved me 'til death us do part.

An acquaintance I knew a few years ago, to whom I revealed a bit of my story because he was a trained therapist, kept telling me I should just "let it all go." Perhaps he was trying to help, but he didn't understand. Because how can you let go of something that is forever in your body?

PARENTAL CONSENT

My mother did not approve of my marrying Mark, for many reasons. First, it was all happening too fast. We met in March and planned to get married in Sept. or Oct. of 1983. Too much, too fast.

Second, he was Jewish. So while Julian was Christian and black, Mark was Jewish and white. I suppose I couldn't get the combo right to suit my parents' wishes.

Third, she just didn't like Mark.

Of the three warnings, this is the one I should have listened to. My mother really did have a sixth sense about people. Her radar was uncanny when it came to noticing subtle cues about people, clues that the person was not all they seemed to be.

My dad, on the other hand, was surprisingly supportive. When Mark met my parents, he said he was going to take care of me financially. He handed my credit cards back to them and said they never had to worry about my being financially secure. Since my dad really cared about money, that was good enough for him.

My brother and sister tried to be supportive of me even though they, too, had misgivings; they became even more supportive, though, when my mother refused to attend the wedding. Although she eventually changed her mind, that period of time was really difficult for me. Here I had found someone who made me happy — or so I thought — and my own mother was making me feel miserable.

Later on, my mother had no idea what was going on in our household the whole time Mark and I were married, up until about two months before I finally walked out. For nearly seven years, I hid it from everyone. Everyone. Maybe I didn't want to admit I had made a mistake. I was definitely embarrassed.

Who wants to admit that their husband is violent? Because, after all, you're still in the marriage with him! What does that say about you, the target of the violence? How weak must you be to stay with someone like that?

Eventually, we had the wedding, Oct. 22, 1983. Everyone was there, including my mother. And the next day, my new husband became someone I didn't recognize.

FIRST SIGN OF TROUBLE

I saw Mark's temper only once before we were married: when I told him in June of 1983 that we couldn't get a September date for our wedding — the church didn't have any openings until October.

I've thought about that moment often, which happened at his sister Lynn's apartment.

It was summertime, and Mark and I were planning to use the pool at Lynn's apartment complex. Lynn lived in a rather run-down building, typical for the San Fernando Valley in LA: a small, U-shaped complex, two stories with outdoor hallways, a front gate that led to mailboxes, a pool in the center of everything, lots of cement, no plants or greenery to speak of.

But the people who lived in the complex were generally nice, and she lived near a really good Jewish bakery. So we saw Lynn on the weekends and often stayed there overnight. She had a great dog, too, and we enjoyed taking him for walks.

I had received the phone call from the church on a Friday,

and I met Mark at Lynn's apartment Saturday morning — a rare Saturday when Mark wasn't working. It always smelled like coffee in Lynn's place. Not liking coffee myself, the smell always made me feel slightly sick.

When I told Mark about the "postponement" (we had wanted to get married in September), he didn't get mad at me, actually. He just got mad in general, and said, loudly, "I don't want to wait until October!"

Then he kicked the screen door at his sister's apartment and bent it off the frame. Lynn was a little bent out of shape that he wrecked her screen door. He promised to pay for it and have it replaced.

At the time, even though his temper outburst surprised me, I thought, Well, everyone gets mad sometimes. No big deal. But obviously, I didn't take it as seriously as I should have.

BACK FROM THE HONEYMOON

While Mark and I were on our honeymoon, my family decorated our apartment so that it looked beautiful when we returned. They had bought some new drapes and a few things for the kitchen and bathroom.

Our gifts were stacked lovingly on the dining room table, which had fresh flowers on it. And in the bedroom was a gorgeous quilt that my friend's mother had made for us.

When we walked in and saw all of this, Mark feigned happiness about it. I was devastated.

On what should have been a glorious, lovely occasion, returning from my honeymoon with my new husband to our cute apartment, I felt like crying. I remember feeling like I just didn't know what to do. Frozen.

Believe me, I know what many people would think: Why didn't you just leave, right then?

It's not that simple. Once violence has taken hold of you, and you're suddenly in panic mode all the time, you're not thinking clearly. At all. Especially when the perpetrator of that violence is your new husband, who, before the wedding, seemed perfectly normal.

I still remember that quilt, with giant blue flowers on it: like a sad garden. So why did I stay?

I have asked myself that question many times. It's the question society asks of women who stay in abusive relationships.

I have an answer, but I also have another question: Why does he hurt her?

Isn't that the real question we should be asking? Why are men (mostly men) abusing their wives/girlfriends?

I don't have an answer to that, so I will answer the other question.

I stayed because in that first moment of being victimized, when I was raped by my husband on our wedding night, my whole being, my whole self, went into another zone. Suddenly, it was all about staying alive, nothing more, nothing less. And in that zone, you have to make split-second choices every single moment of every single day. It's not an easy "place" to live 24 hours a day, 7 days a week.

Not only does being in this strange self-preservation zone cloud your thinking, but it also makes you keenly aware of what is safe to do and what isn't, and when.

I have read statistics that show a woman's chances of being harmed by her violent partner increase dramatically after she leaves. So it's not as simple as just walking out the door.

I have never been physically harmed by a stranger. But imagine for just a moment, God forbid, that you have been raped by a stranger. Only this stranger knows your name, where you live, what you like to eat and drink, knows your family and where they live, knows your birth date, has keys to your home and your car, knows where you work, what you like to do for fun, and on and on.

How safe would you feel just walking away and not making contingency plans, since this guy knows everything about you?

My guess is, not very.

There are many, many reasons why women stay. For me, it wasn't economic, because I knew I could support myself. In my case, it was partly religious, in that I felt that marriage was sacred, and I vowed to remain committed to my husband. But it really was about fear. I was horribly, irrevocably afraid that Mark would kill me. I saw it in his eyes during that first rape. If he could rape me, his bride, on our wedding night, I knew he was capable of anything.

COUNSELOR NO. 1

I went to see a counselor just three months after Mark and I were married.

I knew something was wrong. That may seem obvious, painfully obvious. But because of the state of shock and denial I was in, I couldn't articulate what, exactly, was wrong.

I can't quite remember how I found her, but Laura was a nice woman, a marriage, family and child counselor (MFCC). She held her sessions in her home, which was comfortable but noisy — she lived, literally, next to the freeway. She explained that they were just renting the place and living there temporarily, and they had learned to tolerate the loud hum of traffic.

At that time, Laura was probably 40 years old or so, sort of a motherly figure since I was only 22. She was kind, and she listened to me explain that my brand-new marriage was "off," and I didn't know what to do about it.

I remember telling her that I did not want to be intimate

with Mark, but I never told her exactly why — I tried to block the initial rape and subsequent abuse from my mind, and I was not going to volunteer anything like that to Laura.

That was the problem. Laura never asked me, not once, if I was afraid of Mark, or if he had ever hurt me or tried to hurt me. All of the therapy focused on me, on whatever problems Laura determined me to have, like "mild depression" and fears of intimacy.

I remember telling her that I didn't want Mark to touch me, to the point where if I found one of his hairs in the shower, it completely grossed me out. Her response was, "Can't you think of a hair as a small part of Mark that's with you, even when he's not physically present? It's a token reminder that he's always with you."

That comment made me feel nothing but guilt, like there was something wrong with me for feeling this way.

I do blame Laura for not being more inquiring, not being more observant of my behavior. Maybe I had already gotten very good at hiding my fear of Mark, I don't know. In my own way, I was trying to reach out to someone, but Laura didn't pick up on that at all. I was the one with the problem. Not Mark.

NO DRINKING, NO DRUGS

I wish I could blame Mark's behavior on drinking or drugs. It simply wasn't the case. He never did drugs, and the most I ever saw him drink in one sitting was half a beer. Because his work involved physical labor, he was health conscious and ate very well.

No, the reasons behind Mark's behavior are still rather a mystery to me. What made him feel like I had to obey him, that I couldn't be my own person? That I had to be controlled and manipulated by violence and threats?

I have no definitive answers to those questions.

Mark's family was extremely dysfunctional. Many years later, I came to learn that there was, most likely, incest in the family when he was growing up, which did not completely surprise me. His mother suffered from severe depression, no doubt either brought on or exacerbated by his father's controlling and abusive personality. His sisters were, sadly, train wrecks: drugs, abusive or unhealthy relationships, an inability to take care of themselves financially, lack of education.

But Mark himself was well educated, smart and capable. He had a lot going for him, a lot he could feel proud of. That he continually had to try and keep me in my place — well, I still don't understand why. I can't just write him off as "evil," because to me, it seemed like everything he did was a conscious choice.

Perhaps counseling would have helped him, perhaps not. He continues, to this day, to assert that nothing happened.

I beg to differ.

COUNSELOR NO. 2

During my marriage to Mark, I saw another counselor who came highly recommended by a friend of ours. Bob was a full-fledged psychologist with a fancy office in Century City, a major corporate and shopping hub in LA.

Bob had the same opinion as counselor no. 1, Laura, although at least Laura seemed to listen to me. Bob spent most of his time sitting back in his chair, fidgeting and looking at the 180-degree view out his top-floor window.

Yes, Bob, too, said that I was "mildly depressed" and had problems with intimacy. As they say, No shit, Sherlock.

Bob never asked me if anything had happened during our marriage that would make me afraid of Mark. He never asked if Mark yelled at me, physically harmed me or abused me in any way.

It may seem hard to believe that I wouldn't bring up these issues on my own. The reality is, though, that when you are living in an abusive relationship every day, you slowly close yourself off from reality. Your whole life becomes centered around staying safe by anticipating your partner's every move. Being so focused on another person obliterates your focus on yourself.

You become blind to what you think, feel, need or want. It's always about the other person.

At the time, I had never heard the words "domestic violence" before. I had never personally known anyone — or at least I wasn't aware of anyone — who had been in that type of situation. It was the antithesis of how I grew up and how my past relationships had been.

Mark knew I saw these counselors, and he thought it was a good idea — to fix whatever was wrong with me.

WALKING ON BROKEN GLASS

When I try to think of an analogy about living with a violent spouse, I consistently come back to an image of a woman walking on broken glass.

The woman is clothed, but barely: the shards have torn her clothing apart over time. She is smiling, and her face is smeared with blood, as are her arms, legs and feet.

As she walks across the glass, she grimaces slightly but keeps smiling, never saying a word about the pain she must be feeling.

Her feet are so torn up by the glass, she can't walk very fast, and she certainly can't run anywhere. With every step, she knows she risks being hurt. But she must walk through her day, and her life, so she treads carefully. Without even making a true misstep — because, of course, the glass is everywhere and unavoidable — she still manages to get hurt.

Some of the cuts are deep, some aren't, but they all cause pain. Nothing she does — no way that she walks, or talks, or moves — can change the fact that she will be hurt by the broken glass under her feet.

Soon, because she's spent so much time navigating the glass, the shards become part of her. The pieces that were once strewn about the floor, over time, start to disappear. Her feet absorb them, first the tiny pieces, and then even the large ones find a home inside her. Instead of cutting her on the outside, now the glass really becomes dangerous: it's tearing her apart from the inside.

And since the glass is now part of her, she no longer feels the pain in quite the same way. She still feels the fear of being cut, but now, she's almost doing it to herself. If only I hadn't walked on all that glass in the first place, I wouldn't be in this situation. It's my own fault, she thinks — even though it was her husband, not her, who broke the glass all over the floor.

But it's too late. She *is* the broken glass.

I KNOW WHAT THE QUESTIONS ARE

People's usual questions:

- Why does she stay with him? Why doesn't she just leave? or
- Why did she stay with him for so long?

People's usual answers (who have never been in this situation):

- If my husband did that to me, I would leave him, right then and there.
- I would walk out the door after the very first time.
- She must have low self-esteem.
- She must be uneducated.
- She must think that's how husbands are supposed to treat their wives.
- She must be poor.

- If my husband ever hit me, I would hit him right back.

By the time the reader reaches the end of this book, I hope they will understand why …

1) those are the wrong questions, and 2) those are the wrong answers.

MIND GAMES

I am genuinely paranoid about losing or misplacing important paperwork. Honestly, I'm not using the word "paranoid" lightly. It truly is an irrational fear of mine.

Mark wasn't just sexually, physically and verbally abusive. He also played mind games with me.

One of his favorites was making me think I had lost something valuable or important, usually paperwork related to the house or to his business. He would rush up to me and ask me what I did with his papers/invoices/receipts/whatever it was. When I would say I didn't know what he was talking about, his eyes would widen, his voice would get louder, and he'd try to physically intimidate me. He'd get in my face and raise his arms in the air over his head, as if he were literally going to pound me into the ground.

I didn't touch his paperwork, ever. But he insisted that when I cleaned house, I must be moving things around or putting papers away somewhere.

Within seconds, he'd have me believing that I had, in fact, lost his important papers. So in a panic, I would stop whatever I was doing and rush through the house, searching for whatever it was that he lost.

Only it turns out, he never actually lost anything. He always knew where it was, whatever "it" happened to be. After a few minutes of my scrambling and running around in circles and scared to death he was going to knock my block off, he would magically find the lost item. But then he'd blame me, anyway.

To this day, I hate dealing with any sort of paperwork. I'm terrified I will lose something that is irreplaceable, that will screw up my taxes, or get me in trouble with the bank, the mortgage holder, my employer, or whomever. This fear overtakes me a lot of the time, and when I actually do misplace something, the terror that strikes my chest is physically painful.

It is one thing in my life I desperately want to gain control over. Nothing I have ever done has seemed to mitigate it.

BROKEN MEMORIES

There are many incidents of abuse of which I have only fragmented memories. I will remember the beginning, the middle or the end, but not everything at the same time.

I remember falling hard against the floor in the bedroom and hitting my head when I landed. Just before that, I remember a flash of being on the bed, or perhaps sort of bouncing off of it. I'm spinning, and suddenly I'm on the floor, head first.

Mark is in the room, yelling obscenities as I try to regain my senses. I can hear him saying something like, "I should just go find myself a prostitute!" He would often threaten me with that kind of language if I refused to have sex with him, so I imagine that this falling-on-my-head incident happened after one of my attempts at refusal.

Even now, though, I can re-create in my mind that feeling of being spun to the ground by someone shoving me so hard that I actually flew across the room. I remember looking up from the navy-blue carpeted floor at the wallpaper that I so carefully chose: a beautiful shade of blue-gray and a sort of peach/tan accent, in a soothing abstract pattern.

Strange, the things we remember — and forget.

SCREAMING

Right now, I can hear a guy outside screaming and swearing at someone. He won't stop. So I just raised my window and yelled, "Shut up!" at the top of my lungs. Didn't faze him. He didn't even look in my direction, even though I could see him clearly. He's probably mentally ill. It looked like he was snooping through garbage. But there was another guy with him, sitting on a concrete barrier nearby, so he wasn't screaming and swearing at the voices in his own head — at least, I don't think so.

One after-effect of the violence I experienced — maybe it's part of post-traumatic stress disorder, PTSD — is that I have zero tolerance for screaming, especially when it's combined with swearing. The worst is if it's all directed at someone else, not me.

This is a rather significant problem, especially because I now live in a big city and come into contact with people every day who scream and swear at each other, at their kids, at mass transit when it breaks down, at no one in particular.

Screaming/swearing is one thing that I physically and emotionally cannot tolerate. My mind shuts down, like a steel door slamming shut and plunging me into darkness. My body shuts down, numb and blank. I start to shake. I've learned to control the shaking so that the outside world can't see it. But my whole body, from the inside out, shakes uncontrollably, as if I'm going into shock.

The man outside has stopped his shouting. He has moved on. I am still shaking. I haven't been able to move on.

LAST GLIMPSE OF JULIAN

After I married Mark and my life, overnight, became such a nightmare, all I wanted to do was go back in time and try to fix my relationship with Julian.

I had dreams of him showing up at the church and whisking me away, like in the movie The Graduate.

I saw Julian a couple of times while I was married. One I remember particularly vividly. At the time, I was considering a career in sound engineering, like for musical artists. In the sound-engineering course I was taking, we were allowed to bring in a band, if we knew one, and help them produce/record a piece of music.

So I got in touch with Julian, who was still playing in a band with my friend Scott and some other friends, and brought them into the studio.

It was so much fun for me — like the old days of going to Julian's band rehearsals and hanging out with all our friends.

The session went sort of late, like around midnight. Afterward, Julian and I talked for a short while out in the parking lot. All we did was talk. It was difficult for both of us — me, because I was trying not to let on how miserable I was in my marriage; and him, because I had really hurt him by ending the relationship.

When we drove away from the studio, we each merged onto the freeway, with my car in front of his. He purposely drove very, very slowly, so after a few minutes, I couldn't help but pull away from him. I kept looking in the rear-view mirror for his car, until the last glimpse of his Mustang faded from view.

I pulled up to Mark's and my apartment and parked on the street. Immediately, I knew something was wrong, because the lights were on.

Mark was sitting in the dining room, holding a gift a dear friend of mine had made for me: a glass candy jar on which she had hand etched my name.

Mark threw it at me.

I ducked and it missed me, but it shattered into a thousand pieces.

He was angry that I was out so late, and I guess he suspected something had happened with Julian and me — I had been honest and told him that Julian and his band were coming into the studio.

After he screamed for a minute, he went to bed. I cleaned up the mess. I then proceeded to decorate the dining room for two or three hours with handmade "I'm sorry, forgive me" signs and crepe paper that I saved from another party.

In the morning, he said nothing about the night before or the decorations. I left them up for the rest of the day.

NEVER

When I was a kid, I never heard my parents argue. Never. Not once.

Maybe they did, and I just wasn't around to hear it, I don't know. But I never heard either of my parents raise their voices to each other or to me. They might have discussed things intently at times, and I certainly felt tension between them occasionally. But no one yelled or screamed or caused a scene.

And never, ever did anyone raise a hand to anyone in our household.

We never even had alcohol in the house (not because of religious beliefs), so no one ever got drunk (no smoking, either).

I think it's why I went into an immediate state of shock when Mark first hurt me, because it was a completely new experience for me. I don't mean that glibly; it's a fact. The first time you get physically assaulted — God forbid it should ever happen — it's quite a shock. Especially when the abuser is someone who, just hours before, vowed in front of 100 people to honor and cherish you.

My instant reaction was self-preservation, and fighting back was clearly not an option with him. Remaining passive was the only thing I could do to save my life. It's hard to explain, except that when you look into another person's eyes, and their whole being has suddenly become consumed by rage while they have you in their grip, physically trying to fight them seems like the worst choice.

In that moment on our wedding night when he raped me, I really thought Mark might kill me if he had the chance. His anger was palpable, like a fever had overtaken him. I had never seen anything like that before, and it terrified me.

Terrified me.

I lived in that state of terror for decades: seven years of marriage, and for many more years after I finally moved out.

WANTING A BABY

When I was growing up, my parents didn't offer me any real guidance when it came to going to college or choosing a career. Although they paid for my college education, they never asked me about what I was learning or talked with me about what I might want to do with my life.

I often wonder if things had been different, if I'd been infused with just a little bit of confidence by my parents, I would have chosen to marry Mark. As it was, I often felt put down by my father, in particular, who always seemed to find fault with me. He'd look at a high school report card with five A's and one B+, and the first thing he'd say was, "What happened in that class?"

Even though I had no ideas about a possible career, I always knew I wanted to be a mother. From a very young age, I imagined myself caring for a baby, loving a child, and raising him or her to adulthood.

After four years of marriage to Mark, I suddenly decided it was time to have that child I dreamed of. Looking back on that decision now, I realize that I simply could not picture myself ever being out of that marriage – so, no time like the present, as they say.

I've learned, through intensive counseling, that this inability to envision the future – or a different future – is extremely common among people who have suffered serious trauma, especially protracted trauma like domestic violence. I imagine, then, that I thought I was going to be married to Mark forever and had no choice but to have a child with him, as opposed to being married and having children with someone else, someone who wasn't abusive.

So I got pregnant.

During the pregnancy, Mark was – shockingly – decent. He stopped harassing me, he stopped demanding sex, and he generally behaved like a more normal husband. He wasn't exactly loving toward me, but I could pretend for a while that everything was OK.

I had some problems during the pregnancy, though. I was terribly nauseated for the first three months and was plagued by horrific nightmares. Most nights during my pregnancy, I dreamed about dismembered babies, their limbs floating in space and their faces wide eyed and screaming.

At seven months, I went into premature labor while also having a problem with one of my kidneys, which swelled up to twice its normal size. After several days in the hospital in the ICU, I was released and was given powerful medication to stop the labor.

Fortunately, the baby stayed where she belonged until it was time to come into the world.

"ANOTHER BITCH"

***

It's the morning after my daughter was born. I am recovering in the hospital but so very happy to have her in my arms. Being a mother has been the only thing in my life that I've ever really felt comfortable doing. It started the day she was born, that feeling of "this is what I was meant to do with my life."

Mark is in the room with me, and a few of his family members have come to meet little Sarah. Mark is the youngest of four children and has three older sisters. At this particular moment, it was one of his male relatives who had come to visit — I can't remember if it was a cousin or a brother-in-law, but I do remember that it was not his father.

So this man, whoever he was, comes into the room and says, "Mark, you have a daughter!" To which Mark replies, "Yes. Another bitch. Another bitch in the family."

At that very moment, I was emotionally flung back to our wedding night when he raped me. Shock. Hurt. Even deeper this time, if that's possible. How could I, or anyone, accept that a man could say something like that about his infant daughter, not even 24 hours old?

The man chuckled a little, perhaps out of nervousness. It had been a good nine months for me, free from Mark's abuse. But it started again that very day, with that comment about my beautiful, beautiful Sarah.

TWO WHOLE WEEKS

After I gave birth to Sarah, Mark refused to allow anyone in my family to come see us for two weeks. Two whole weeks. They lived within seven hours' driving distance, and he refused to have them visit us.

I tried not to let it bother me, but it was so very painful not to see my mother, especially, after giving birth. I wanted to share those first few days with her. As it turned out, my mother died when Sarah was just 3 years old — and I grieve for the time that we could have shared, once in a lifetime.

I sometimes wonder why my family didn't suspect that something was terribly wrong. This was not the first time Mark had denied their visits. Perhaps I became adept at making up excuses. I certainly am not blaming anyone, especially my family, for my situation. I do wonder, though, how the marriage looked from the outside. When I look at photographs of myself from those years, I am terribly thin, thinner than I should have been. I barely recognize myself.

During those first two weeks of Sarah's life, I was really on my own. Mark didn't take any time off from work — he had his own business — so I did everything. He occasionally changed a diaper, and he liked to play with Sarah and talk to her. But I remember not having much time to recuperate before having to do all the normal chores, like going to the supermarket, cleaning the house, cooking, and the like. About three days after giving birth, I asked Mark if he would please go pick up the photos that were taken during delivery – they were ready. He told me I could go myself. So I put Sarah in the car, drove to the photo place, and picked them up, walking slowly and gingerly to avoid the discomfort from the massive amount of stitches I unfortunately required.

Despite everything, though, I really took to parenting. Like every new parent, there were times when I wasn't exactly sure what Sarah needed. But I read a lot, and I listened to the pediatrician's suggestions about nursing and whatnot, and things fell into place with the baby.

Mark stayed fairly calm for about six months or so after Sarah was born. But then, the real Mark appeared once again, worse than ever.

IN THE PRESENT TENSE

⚜

It is nighttime. I am in Hawaii, on Maui. My daughter is 6 months old, and she is sleeping in a portable crib in the bedroom of the rented condo. My sister-in-law is in the condo next door — or rather, that's where she's staying, but she's out partying, as usual, even though we paid her way here so she could baby sit.

Mark wants me to give him a blow job.

His temper is always at its peak whenever we go on vacation.

I hesitate. I don't say no – in fact, I say nothing – but I hesitate.

Suddenly I feel a hand around my throat. I see his wide hazel eyes staring at me with hatred in them, burning, flashing with anger. I see snarling teeth, and I hear a voice becoming agitated, though quietly so as not to wake the baby. The voice comes through the teeth. I see the other hand, the one that isn't around my throat, pulled back into a fist. I tune in to the voice for a few seconds, but the room is starting to spin. *Break your teeth*, I hear. *Break your teeth.*

I'm not really hearing now. Not really seeing. Stars in front of my eyes, sparkling like the Maui sky. Waves rushing into my ears, underwater sounds enveloping me. Nighttime enters my mind. I'm floating somewhere.

And then suddenly, the light starts to come back to my eyes. I feel no more hand on my throat. I gasp a couple of times, and I cough but try not to wake the baby. Cough quietly.

As the light begins to flood my eyes again, I see Mark walk away and I hear a door slam. I cry. I hurt and I cry, quietly.

I wait.

I hear the door open again. It is a few minutes later, I think. Mark walks into the bedroom and takes off his pants.

I give him a blow job. The baby doesn't wake up.

THE DEEPEST GRIEF

I grieve for so many things that I lost because of Mark's abuse. Some are obvious – my youth, my trust in other people, my innocence and exuberance about life.

Some are not obvious to anyone but me.

The deepest grief I feel has to do with being a mother. For when I became Sarah's mother, I really wasn't myself. That self who dreamed of being a mommy someday was gone, never to be seen again. The self that replaced her was someone who was emotionally frozen inside a traumatic and violent relationship, struggling every day to stay alive and, now, to protect a baby from Mark.

How could she ever be the mother she hoped to be, under those circumstances? How could she ever feel even one moment of peace to focus solely on herself or her child?

The answer is: She couldn't. I couldn't.

My role as mother, the only I role ever really wanted in my life, was stained and ruined forever by the abuse Mark perpetrated on me. I did not consciously know that at the time. But I certainly see it clearly now.

How might I have been a different mother? In more ways that I can even fathom. I would have been a better example of a professional person, with a career -- since I have never had one. More importantly, I would have been excited about life, energetic and at the same time, relaxed and focused on motherhood and on Sarah.

So many emotions are tied to motherhood, and mothers do so much for their children out of love. If I had been allowed -- Mark would not let me do these things -- I would have made some clothes for her, learned to knit blankets for her, played music and taught her the piano. It was so ingrained in me that I was never supposed to do those things, ever again, that even when Sarah got older and I had left the marriage, I never did them. The things in life that used to give me joy, to this day make me feel guilty for doing them. Because with Mark, anything that took my focus off of him was forbidden, implicitly and explicitly.

"You cannot play the piano when I'm at home."

"You may not use the sewing machine unless it's to repair my clothes."

Of all the losses, I feel this one the most deeply. I can never, ever go back and be the mother I could have been, should have been, deserved to be.

After I had Sarah, I did not go back to my old job. Mark and I had agreed that I would stay home with her until she started school.

Within the tormented existence — truly, just an existence

— I had with Mark, I tried to create some sort of life for Sarah and me, even without some of life's pleasures.

After Mark left for work in the morning, usually by 7 a.m., I had the day to be with my daughter. I remember those days as a time of respite, where I could feel a bit like myself again. I could take care of this beautiful child, and in turn nourish myself with all that she gave me in return. Even though the time we had was fleeting, because Mark would always come home, I tried to use the time to its fullest extent.

The specter of Mark was always there, but even so, I enjoyed being a new mom. Nursing went well, and I became known as "earth mother" because I used cloth diapers (that I washed myself) and made baby food instead of buying it in the jars. It all felt very natural to me. It helped that Sarah was an easygoing baby who slept and ate well.

I tried to shield her from the other life – the existence. I took more blows, literally and figuratively, from Mark in order to keep him away from Sarah.

Eventually, I realized I couldn't really protect her. And worst of all, I hadn't protected her.

BLURTING IT OUT

⚜

Mark and I spent a lot of time with his family, in particular his cousin Josh and his wife (and their children, eventually). Josh and his wife were Orthodox, and we often went to their home for dinner Friday night.

I enjoyed their company. Out of all the members of Mark's family, they seemed the most normal, the most "together." Josh was a doctor, a good one, and was very engaging; his wife, Naomi, was an artist with a lot of energy and enthusiasm for life. We had some very good discussions about politics, religion and Israel, and even though Mark had cut me off from my other friends over time, I felt like Josh and Naomi were my friends.

One time, several months after Sarah was born, Josh and Naomi were at our house. We were sitting in our screened-in room, and as usual it was a beautiful day. Mark had stepped out — I think he went to the store to get something, but in any case, he wasn't home.

I was talking with Josh and Naomi, but I wasn't focused at all on the conversation at hand. The entire time, I was trying to get up my nerve to tell them about Mark's behavior, and to ask for their help. This really was the first time I even thought about asking anyone for help. Being that Josh was a doctor, I thought he might be receptive to what I was going to say, even though I was going to criticize Mark.

When I realized I was running out of time and that Mark would be home any minute, I blurted it out, in the middle of the conversation: "Mark's temper gets really out of control. Sometimes he can be violent and abusive toward me, and now I'm afraid he might hurt Sarah."

I remember feeling an overwhelming sense of panic as I spoke, and the words fell from my mouth. I am sure I turned white, because my heart was racing and the room started to spin.

Josh and Naomi just sat there, staring at me. Then they looked at each other for an uncomfortable moment, saying nothing but looking a bit unnerved.

It couldn't have been more than 30 seconds, when Mark suddenly came home.

I thought, certainly Josh and Naomi care about me and Sarah, and they'll find a way to talk to me later; maybe they'll call or invite me over to their house.

Nothing. I never heard a word. I was devastated, and looking back, I think that one experience stopped me from asking for help until I finally reached my ultimate decision to leave.

After I moved out, I never heard from Josh and Naomi again.

A JAB IN THE BACK CAN BE A GOOD THING

My best friend Kim doesn't realize it — I have never shared it with her — but a gesture she made to me was one of the final clues that told me I had to leave Mark.

Kim and I were in a playgroup together and had actually known each other since we were college age. She was really the only friend from my pre-Mark days with whom I had any regular contact.

At the time, my daughter was 2, Kim's son going on 3. All around us were other kids and moms, playing some sort of game. To be honest, I never enjoyed the playgroup very much, although it certainly provided some socialization for Sarah. I never felt completely comfortable with the women in the group. Many of them seemed uptight about parenting, and I had to work diligently to keep that worry from rubbing off on me – I had enough problems of my own to worry about. If there was one thing in life I didn't fret over, it was my parenting skills. I wasn't perfect, but I felt confident in my abilities from all the reading I was doing, so I didn't need anyone to instill fear in that particular element of my life.

Kim and I were sitting on the floor during one of the playgroups, hosted at another mom's house. I must have been really slumped over, because she took her thumb and jabbed it into my back, hard, like, Straighten up!

That gesture was telling. I was so emotionally and physically beaten down, I couldn't even sit up straight anymore. And I had just found out I was pregnant again.

When I was pregnant with Sarah, Mark took a nine-month break from the violence. With this second pregnancy, though, the violence escalated. There was no break at all, and I felt seriously endangered. Although I didn't know it at the time, I discovered later than one reason for the escalation of the violence was that Mark was having an affair (probably one of many).

Even though I hadn't consciously thought of leaving at that point, that jab in the back was in my mind a couple of months later, when I did make the decision to walk out the door.

In the year and a half since Sarah had been born, Mark's anger had gradually increased to an unbearable level. Every day brought with it new threats, threats which I bore in order to keep Sarah safe. I was living in total fear and completely overcome by trauma by this point, six years into the marriage.

Mark was not happy about the pregnancy. At all.

He made that very clear one day, about six weeks into the pregnancy.

I was in the laundry room, actually enjoying the chore because the sun was pouring in through the windows. Suddenly Mark burst in, screaming obscenities at me at the top of his lungs. I don't even remember what he was saying. I backed myself against the other wall in a big hurry to try and put some distance between us. Before I knew what was happening, he was up in my face, waving a beer bottle.

As I mentioned, Mark didn't drink or do drugs. He would have about half a beer every other night, but that was it. So he wasn't drunk. I wish I could use that as an excuse for his behavior, but it's not true.

I cannot remember the exact words he was yelling at me, because all I saw was the bottle in his hand and his face in my face. He was holding the bottle up over his head, as though he were going to crack it on my skull. I couldn't take my eyes off of it. The beautiful sunny day and the smell of clean laundry faded to black. All I could think of was how much it was going to hurt to get hit with that bottle. His other hand was to the side of my face, against the wall. There was no escape.

Suddenly, he backed off. He screamed some more at me, and then went out into the back yard with the bottle and threw it on the ground.

I finished the laundry and then went out into the sunlight to sweep up the glass.

A WITNESS

◈

My mother came to visit Mark, Sarah and me in June of 1990. As usual, she stayed in a hotel, even though Mark could have slept on the sofa for a few days or, as I had wanted, we could have bought a guest bed and put it in Sarah's room.

I had recently found out I was pregnant with our second child, and I hadn't yet told my mom. I was waiting for the right moment in her visit to do so, but I couldn't seem to get up the nerve to tell her.

Mark was working a lot. Having his own business, he was in charge of everything, and over the years he had gained some very important and wealthy clients who expected him to be at their beck and call.

We had been having some trouble with the pool, keeping the chemicals balanced. I watched as, day by day, the water became more and more green.

My mom was excellent with pool chemicals, since she had

had a pool for many years. So one morning during her visit, after Mark had left for work, we decided to surprise him by fixing the pool chemicals.

He would come home that night not only to a nice dinner, but also to a sparkling, clear and beautiful pool.

We went to the store and bought all the chemicals, and we came home and started working on it. Within just a few hours, the change in the water was dramatic. By the time Mark came home, the pool looked perfect.

But his reaction was not.

Mark saw the pool and quickly turned on his heels and pulled me into the bedroom. He closed the door and flew into a rage, while my mom stood in the other room, overhearing everything. He was screaming at the top of his lungs, something like, how dare we touch HIS pool and adjust HIS chemicals.

How dare we.

He was so angry, that he jumped up onto the bed and was bouncing up and down, like he was on a trampoline. By that point, I had been able to open the bedroom door, and my mom saw his positively crazy behavior. She was aghast, as she had never seen or heard him act like this. The horror on her face ... I can still visualize it today, her mouth gaping open, her blue-green eyes wide and unblinking.

I told her it was going to be all right, just please go sit in the living room while I calm him down.

Against my better judgment but afraid he might come out and attack my mother, I went back in the bedroom and tried to reason with Mark. He jumped off the bed, grabbed my arm so hard I thought he might break it, and said, softly into my ear through gritted teeth, "You or your mother must leave this house right now, or one of you is going to be dead."

The bruise was forming on my arm. I took his threat seriously.

I quickly took my mother back to her hotel and booked her on a plane back home that very day.

It was one of the hardest things I had ever had to do. Ever.

What did I say to her? I made up excuses about him being under stress or something. And I also told her I was pregnant.

She begged me to be careful, suggested that maybe I should leave, but I told her it was going to be OK, that she shouldn't worry.

I remember waving good bye to her at the airport, and I went back to the car and cried for 15 minutes before driving back to the house, all the time wondering if Mark was going to hurt me again or if he had calmed down.

When we got home, he said nothing.

My mother was the only person who ever witnessed his behavior.

MISCARRIAGE

I am playing the piano, rehearsing one of the songs from "Phantom of the Opera" to perform at my sister- in-law's wedding in a few days. The singer is one of her colleagues. Her voice is so-so, passable, I guess.

I'm doing my best to accompany her well and support her vocal strengths and hide her weaknesses.

It's now time for her to leave. When I stand up from the piano bench, I feel something wet between my legs. As graciously as possible, I escort her to the door, and after seeing her off, I run to the bathroom.

Blood. Bright red blood.

I'm 11 weeks pregnant.

Mark and Sarah are at the beach and are due home soon. I decide not to wait for them, and I call my doctor, who tells me to meet him at the hospital.

As I drive myself there, I repeat over and over again, a

hundred times, "God is in control of this. God is in control of this."

After I arrive at the hospital, I meet my doctor who does an exam, and a technician does an ultrasound. "It's the beginning of a miscarriage," my doctor tells me. He suggests I go home and wait until things progress a bit more before coming back to the hospital. I'm not sure exactly what he means by that, but I do what he says.

When I get home, Mark is there. I'd left him a note, explaining what was going on. We try to make the rest of the day as normal as possible, for Sarah's sake. But Mark doesn't seem all that upset about what's happening.

I go to bed at 10 pm.

At 11 pm, I wake up in agony. Suddenly, it feels like I'm laboring at about 6 cm. I don't say anything to Mark — I don't wake him up.

I go into the bathroom, and for several hours, I sit on the toilet and experience the horror that is a miscarriage. Blood, pieces of placenta, my pregnancy ... my beautiful baby ... flows out of me into the bowl.

At about 5 am, I am in even more pain than before. I think something must be wrong in addition to the miscarriage. I wake Mark and ask him to drive me to the ER. So we wake 2-year-old Sarah, put her in the car seat and drive to the hospital.

I'm escorted to one of the curtained "rooms" in the ER, and I wait, and wait, and wait for the doctor. And I cry. A nurse, as she's reading my chart, asks why I'm crying.

I "complete" the miscarriage in the ER, and my doctor explains that I need a D&C to make sure nothing was left behind.

By this point, I am emotionally and physically numb already. No anesthetic needed, I think to myself.

As I'm about to be wheeled to the operating room, Mark doesn't say anything to me. He doesn't say he's sorry about what's happened. He doesn't seem sad or upset at all.

The nurse says to him, curtly, "Your wife is about to have a procedure done, under general anesthetic. Don't you want to say good bye to her and give her a kiss?"

He says good bye as he walks away down the hall to meet his mother, who has come to help with Sarah. Mark and Sarah drive home in his mom's car while I have my D&C.

I wake up from the anesthetic and am taken to a hospital room. There is no one in the waiting room for me, so I spend the next couple of hours alone, watching TV.

I call my mother and tell her what happened, but I don't dramatize it. She lost a baby, too — at five months' gestation — so she doesn't need to be reminded of the emotional pain it causes.

After they've determined I'm OK to leave, I drive myself home, since our car is still in the parking lot.

Sarah is in the back yard with her grandma when I arrive at the house, and Mark is in the living room. I don't say anything to him. I go into Sarah's room, where I had already started arranging a few things for the new baby, and I crumple to the floor in a rush of tears.

Mark doesn't say anything or come over to me. Instead, he goes into our bedroom. "I need you!" I scream, as he shuts the door behind him.

I pick up a red wooden building block and throw it against the wall. It leaves a permanent dent.

DINNER PLATE

◈

Since much of Mark's work involved physical labor, he had to eat well. He also was hypoglycemic (undiagnosed, as he hated going to the doctor), so his blood sugar was highly affected by what he ate and when.

In preparing dinner every night, I tried to consider what he needed in order to be able to do his work. I experimented with a lot of different recipes, and I became a fairly good cook. He, too, enjoyed cooking and was very inventive in the kitchen.

One time, I remember him having a particularly rough week in terms of work — very, very busy, and very hard physical labor. I decided I would make him a delicious steak dinner, with all the trimmings: good vegetables, baked potatoes, the works.

When he came home that night, he quickly took a shower while I finished preparing dinner. After his shower, he came into the kitchen to see what I was making. Sarah was playing in the family room, and we had a small pass-through opening from the kitchen to the family room to hand things back and forth, if needed.

He asked what I made, and I proudly handed him a dinner plate filled with gorgeous food: a perfectly cooked steak, baked potato with all the toppings he liked, and two vegetables.

Before I knew it, he was in my face, holding the plate over my head.

"Why did you make STEAK for dinner?!" he screamed. "I don't want STEAK for dinner! I already had MEAT for lunch today! Don't you realize by now that I often have meat for lunch? DON'T YOU KNOW THAT?"

In an instant, he threw the plate through the pass-through, and it crashed onto a glass coffee table. Miraculously, only the plate broke, but the food was strewn everywhere.

Sarah just happened to be on the opposite side of the room.

I felt a surge of anger but controlled it. "You could have hit Sarah with that," I said as calmly as I possibly could.

"Go get me something else for dinner!" he replied.

I quickly gathered Sarah and went to the car. I got in the car, put her in her car seat (she was about 18 months old), and felt myself shaking. I took a deep breath and drove to the supermarket, thinking, What can I make? What can I make?

We got to the store, and I quickly bought a pre-cooked chicken and some salad. I rushed through the checkout, then back home. I'm surprised I didn't get a speeding ticket.

Once we got home, I prepared the meal in about five minutes and told Mark his dinner was ready.

"I'm not hungry now," he said, without a hint of anger, as I handed him the plate of food. And then he dumped the chicken dinner, plate and all, in the trash.

SAD MOTHER-IN-LAW

Mark's mother, Abigail, was a very nice woman. When I met her in 1983, she was in her mid-50s, and she was fit and active. She played tennis a lot — Mark and I often played with her on the weekends, and she'd beat both of us routinely. I called her "the human backboard." She was an attractive woman, with lovely dark hair flecked with gray, bright and sparkly eyes and a nice smile.

But something was wrong.

Mark had explained early in our relationship that his mother had been hospitalized a few times for severe depression. Although he didn't come right out and say so, he hinted that she had tried to commit suicide, perhaps more than once.

Over the nearly seven years that Mark and I were married, while I was enduring the hell that is domestic violence, I believe Abigail was, too. Mark's father, Gerard, was (is — he's still living) a controlling and scary figure in his own right. He made it clear who was boss, and while I personally never saw him lift a hand to Abigail, I'm sure now that he did.

I know he exerted his considerable powers of mental and emotional abuse on her — I could see it in her eyes, whenever we were around them. She seemed to grow smaller in his presence, and even her voice lowered when she spoke to him.

During my marriage, I gradually came to see Abigail as … well, as me, several decades down the line. I wondered about the reasons for her depression and hospitalizations.

I have thought back to the psychotherapists I saw during my marriage — I saw three of them — who never, ever asked me if my husband hurt me in any way. Instead, they said I was mildly depressed and had problems with intimacy.

Well, duh.

In 2009, I heard that Abigail had died; she drowned in the bathtub while home alone. Apparently she had begun to have problems with dementia, although I wasn't able to confirm that, since I'm not in direct personal contact with anyone in the family (only a couple of Sarah's cousins are still in touch with Sarah).

The last time I saw Abigail was a few years ago. Sarah was going to spend a couple of days at her cousin's house — basically the only relatives on Mark's side of the family that were still in touch with us. We met the cousin and her mother at a park, and Abigail had come along for the ride, too. She gave Sarah and me each a huge hug. Without saying so, somehow I felt she understood what we had experienced and was trying to communicate that to us non-verbally. It was a powerful moment, and tears came to our eyes.

I wish someone had been there all those years to help Abigail and, of course, to prevent her death in that manner, somehow. I don't think she was truly depressed. I think she was a victim of domestic violence, and no one ever asked her about it.

CROSSING OVER

During my marriage to Mark, I felt blind much of the time. And deaf, too. I was trying to become as small and insulated as possible, so Mark wouldn't have any reason to harm me.

Now, I realize, what happened was that I had crossed over from a place of rational thought and inaction, to a place ruled by panic, fear and self-preservation. There was never a moment when I could relax. Never. Even now, I never fully relax.

When someone tells you, screams at you, on a daily basis, that you're a "fucking cunt" and other such things, accompanied by physical threats — grabbing, shoving, pushing, general throttling — and sexual humiliation, you start to believe what they're saying. And being young and idealistic, I thought that since I married Mark, I had made a commitment, and this is what my life was going to be like. Unless maybe I could change him.

So … I did everything in my power to change myself in

order to stop him from behaving that way. I became a meek and lifeless person who had no interests outside of the home. Most of my friends, including my dear friend Scott, and that group of wonderful people I knew in college, slowly vanished from my life.

For nearly seven years, I couldn't see that the bridge I had crossed went both ways — and if I wanted to, I could simply turn and face the other direction, and walk away.

TURNING POINTS

The turning points that helped me decide to leave Mark came in a tumble during 1990. One was a conversation I had with a mother who belonged to Sarah's playgroup.

I cannot recall the exact details of the incident with Mark — there were so many that they are blurred in my memory. But I recounted it to this other mom, whom I will call Sue, one beautiful summer day in 1980.

Sue was at my house, and our daughters, who were around 2 years old at the time, were playing in the family room. I was standing at my dining room table with some snacks for the kids as Sue emerged from the family room to get the food.

Suddenly, I was possessed with the desire to tell someone about what was going on in my household. I didn't even know Sue all that well, which, in hindsight, seems appropriate. After trying to tell someone with whom I was close — Mark's cousin Josh and his wife — and getting nowhere, talking to an acquaintance was probably logical.

"Sue, can I tell you something? Last night, my husband [fill in the blank — grabbed me, shook me, shoved me, screamed at me, some combination of the above]. Should I be concerned?"

Sue stared at me for a moment with a look of disbelief. Then calmly, she said, "Yes, you should be concerned. I think you should move out, right now. If you need a place to stay, you can stay with me."

I was dumbstruck. I couldn't believe her reaction — it seemed extreme to me. Isn't that ironic? But at the same time, I understood what she was saying. Deep down, something was stirring inside me, moving me to … well, make my move.

I told Sue that I really appreciated what she said, and that I would definitely consider it. That conversation, as brief as it was, became one turning point.

NEWSPAPER

⚘

One Sunday morning, Mark was in the family room reading the LA Times. Sarah and I were in there, too, playing on the floor. My darling girl was so much fun – energetic and bright, with insatiable curiosity and a good, happy nature. Her blue eyes sparkled when she looked at me.

"I want some more coffee," Mark said coldly. He never asked me nicely to get something for him, never said "please" or "thank you."

"I'll get it for you in just a second," I said. Sarah was having fun, and I wanted to let her play a bit more before putting her in the playpen so I could get Mark's coffee.

"I want some more coffee," he repeated, not looking up from the paper. That was my warning.

I heeded it, and I picked Sarah up and put her in the playpen. Thankfully, she didn't cry — she quickly became absorbed in playing with her blocks. I always worried about Mark's temper flaring when Sarah cried, because he didn't have much tolerance for anything that disturbed the peace of his home.

It was his home. Not ours. Certainly not mine.

To get to the kitchen, I had to walk through the doorway and past Mark, who was sitting on the sofa next to the doorway. As I walked by him, I felt a hard SMACK on the side of my face, and my left eye was suddenly on fire. Mark had rolled up the paper and hit me with it, and a sharp paper corner had jabbed me in the eye.

I couldn't help myself.

"I'm not a dog!" I yelled, nearly gagging on the words. "I'm not a dog!"

My heart was pounding with fear, thinking I may have just set myself up for something worse. I rushed into the kitchen and poured his coffee, my eye stinging and running so badly I couldn't even see what I was doing. Tears of pain mixed with tears of anger, but both emotions were subsumed by humiliation.

I gave Mark his coffee, and he said nothing. I was relieved as I went into the bathroom and surveyed my left eye, which was completely bloodshot and had a small cut next to it.

I am nothing but a dog. Part of me actually believed it.

K-Y

This is a really difficult section to write, so I'm going to write it as succinctly as possible. One might wonder why I'm even writing it. Is it even germane to this conversation? For me, it is. Because trauma is tangible. It's not just a concept, or a feeling — it's a bodily experience.

In order to have sex with me, Mark would use K-Y jelly. I simply could never relax with him after our honeymoon … because every time he had sex with me, it was forced. It wasn't like he held me down every time. But I didn't want it. Therefore, it was forcible rape, every time.

To this day, I have a minor mental breakdown every time I go to the gynecologist. I think about anything else when they use the K-Y, and I tend to be quite chatty with the doctor and nurse — anything to keep my mind off the dreaded K-Y.

I even avoid seeing it in the drug store. I can't look at a box of it without feeling physically sick.

FEELING UGLY

When I look at photos of myself when I was married to Mark, from age 22 to age 29, I see a woman who was actually quite pretty. People often asked me if I had ever been a model (nope, not interested back then). I was born with typical California-girl looks: very tall, thin, naturally blond, blue eyed. I still am all of those, just not quite as cute today, 20-plus years later.

But during my 20s, I felt ugly. I fought against it, and I took pride in my appearance: I went to a good hair stylist, I shopped for high-quality clothes and made sure I looked professional while I was working (mostly in the legal field, where dressing well makes a good impression).

Mark never said one nice word to me about how I looked. His remarks were always something like, "Why would you wear that?" Or worse still, I'd get dressed up for something special — a rare occurrence, to be honest — and he would say nothing at all. I'm sure his behavior was intentional, to keep me in my place, if you will. To make me feel less than.

It worked.

Being told that I was ugly — in so many words and in no words at all — has stayed with me. To this day, when I see a photo of myself I sometimes think, I don't look that bad. I wish, instead, that I could think, I look great! I'll keep working on that. I know for it to be genuine, that sentiment has to come from within me, not from other people. I have to believe I'm beautiful.

IN BETWEEN

In between the major episodes of Mark's temper, he could be rather congenial. He was never loving to me, never said kind words or thanked me for anything. But he could be at least somewhat like the man I knew before we were married: funny and fun-loving, interesting to talk to.

The problem was, I never knew how long the "in between" period would last. My guard had to be up — constantly. Even when we entertained his family — which we did quite often, since we had a pool and his family enjoyed using it — and things looked relatively normal from the outside, I was still on guard.

Every moment I was in the kitchen preparing food, for example, I worried about whether he would find the meal satisfactory. I fretted over the cleanliness of the house, whether his laundry was done the way he liked it, or whether I had accidentally moved something of his and he wouldn't be able to find it and would blow up at me.

For me, there never was an "in between." I never could guess what would set off his temper. Believe me, I tried. I tried to find a pattern to his behavior that would allow me to anticipate his temper. But I simply couldn't figure it out.

Every day that passed without an incident of violence or strong language directed at me was a small victory for me. But it was a victory I could only enjoy until the next time I awoke, and had to face another day wondering if we were still "in between."

ON THE SOFA

Many nights, to avoid Mark's sexual advances, I would purposely fall asleep on the family room sofa and come into bed well after he had fallen asleep. Mark went to bed early because he had to leave very early in the morning for work. It finally occurred to me that maybe, over time, I could sort of train him to leave me alone.

Over a period of about a year, I was able to gradually avoid going to bed with him at the same time most nights.

Some nights, he insisted, and he would pressure me into having sex with him. But eventually, those nights became fewer.

All of this took a toll, however. I never had one good night's sleep with Mark in the house, let alone next to me in bed. For nearly seven years, my sleep was anything but restful. I always felt like I literally had to sleep with one eye open, guarding myself from danger that could occur at any moment.

The fatigue only added to the chaos in which I continually

lived: the ever-present threat of violence was heightened by a feeling of physical weakness, generated by my lack of sleep.

I did my best to stay strong by exercising a lot. But the lack of good-quality sleep really hurt my health during those years — physical, emotional and mental health.

Imagine for a moment that you are sleeping next to your rapist every night. You never really sleep. Sarah is Afraid

August of 1990 was a horrific month. The first week, I had the miscarriage at 11 weeks pregnant. Mark offered nothing in terms of his own grief (he felt none, clearly) or in support of mine. I came to believe, in fact, that the incident in the laundry room, where he threatened to break a beer bottle over my head, may have caused the miscarriage — it happened nearly to the day that the doctor said the miscarriage probably began (about four weeks before it actually happened).

It was a hot August evening in Los Angeles, and Sarah and I had had a good day. We went to the park, played with some of her friends, and then had fun in the pool together. Mark had been working, and I knew he'd want a good dinner — something special, since he had been working outdoors in the heat.

I remember cooking salmon on the grill, just the way he liked it.

Mark came home, and Sarah and I were in the kitchen. I was finishing the dinner preparations and just about to put the salmon on the plates when Mark walked into the kitchen.

"What are you DOING?!" he screamed. I replied that I made dinner, that I had grilled some salmon. "You don't know how to grill salmon!" he yelled. "Only I know how to do it right!"

With that, he picked up a plate that was sitting on the counter and smashed it into the sink.

Sarah, who was sitting on the floor, turned white. Her blue eyes — large, to begin with — were bigger than I'd ever seen them. And suddenly, she screamed, louder than I'd ever heard her.

I scooped her up in my arms and took her into her bedroom to calm her down, holding her next to my heart that was beating as fast as a hummingbird's. I gave her her favorite blanket, one my mother knitted for her, and the two of us rocked in the rocking chair for a long time.

Click, went my brain. *I must leave.*

EXISTENCE

My life with Mark was not my life. It was my existence.

I tried to pretend that things were OK. I'd kiss Mark good bye in the morning and give him another kiss when he came home. In my mind, I played games with myself, pretending that I had a husband who loved me, protected me, nurtured me.

In the years before Sarah was born and I was working as a legal secretary, I did my best to be professional and form some friendships, albeit surface ones. I think people liked me and appreciated the quality of my work.

I also tried to be part of Mark's family, although it wasn't easy. They were so different from my own family, in nearly every respect. His father was a threatening force. Although not physically strong or intimidating, he had an air about him that signified his power over the family. Mark's mother was depressed and sad, although she, too, put up a good front. I'm certain she was abused, too.

His three sisters, all of whom were older than Mark, were a mess. None went to college, and none of them had achieved any financial or personal success. The oldest of the three, Carla, was a little strange, but nice and in a marriage that, on the surface, seemed OK but I suspected was abusive (turns out I was right). The middle sister, Lynn, was on drugs a lot of the time, although she had some good qualities and tried to befriend me as best she could. The youngest of the three sisters, Pam, couldn't seem to straighten out her relationships (dating a married man for years, having numerous abortions) until she got married in 1990. Of the three sisters, Pam and I had the worst relationship — we just didn't "get" each other at all.

Because Mark had tried to isolate me from my own family and friends — they simply weren't allowed to come and visit, and he got so agitated when I went out at night with anyone that I simply stopped doing it — I felt alone.

And every day, I fought the intense battle to stay safe, to stay alive: constantly trying to second guess Mark's every move, to anticipate his temper, and when he did explode, to react in such a way that he didn't hurt me even worse.

That's not living. It's existing.

MEXICAN VACATION

Shortly after Mark's sister's wedding in August of 1990, Mark, Sarah and I were supposed to go to Mexico on vacation. We had chosen a resort that had lots of stuff for kids to do — even though Sarah was only 2 years old at the time, we thought there might be something fun for her to do.

For reasons I still cannot explain, Mark's behavior was always worse when we were on vacation. Perhaps it was because he wasn't in his own environment, so he felt even more out of control and, therefore, wanted to exert control. Maybe he thought I had more chances to leave him when we were away, so he asserted his authority even more over me by using threats and physical and emotional violence against me.

After all the small signs of the preceding weeks added up to one large message in my mind, that I simply had to leave him, I knew I couldn't possibly wait until after we got back from this vacation. The thought of going on vacation with him made me literally sick to my stomach. All I could picture were more episodes of violence: more rape, more screaming, more everything. I couldn't do it.

I had to figure out a way to leave. And fast. The vacation was only a few days away, by this point. I knew I had to try and gain control of myself, try to make some quick decisions about where I could go and how I could do it without Mark harming me or Sarah.

Sarah. She was first and foremost in my mind, always. I wanted to keep her safe. Keeping calm proved difficult, as I packed my suitcase for the trip to Mexico — with my bathing suit and other beachwear on top, and my real clothes hidden underneath: things I would need right away once Sarah and I had made our escape.

WHO TO TURN TO

When I made the decision to leave Mark, there was no going back. It was a final decision. But I really didn't know who to turn to.

I thought about going to my parents' house, but I didn't feel safe doing that — because Mark knew where they lived. As emotional as I was about this decision, and as much as I was still in shock and trauma from seven years of abuse, I knew I was making a potentially dangerous move. It was one reason I didn't leave long before then.

As the day approached, Aug. 31, 1990, I grew more and more steadfast in my decision. And I made another one: I decided to call Julian.

I had not seen or spoken to Julian in ages, mostly because he had been terribly hurt by our break-up and, of course, Mark would have been insane with jealousy -- even though I never even looked at another man or thought about an affair. I had heard through my best friend Kim, who had also been friends with Julian during college and sometimes had contact with him, that he wasn't married and was having a successful career. I don't remember how I got his number, except that I probably just dialed 4-1-1, like we used to do in those days.

If I were to try and reconstruct the conversation I had with him, which happened two or three days before I left Mark, it would probably look something like a tornado. My mind and emotions were all over the place: disjointed, broken, swirling in a massive funnel cloud inside my head.

I remember that we talked, literally, for hours at a time over a couple of days, all while Mark was working. I remember trying to watch Sarah at the same time I was having these intense conversations and finding myself weeping into the dark blue carpeting on our family room floor while she played nearby.

Over all those hours, I told Julian everything that had been happening in my marriage to Mark. Although he must have been completely overwhelmed, he listened and consoled me, and offered to help in any way he could. Julian suggested that I contact some other friends of ours whom Mark didn't know well and who lived out of town, as a possible place for my escape.

My body literally shook with fear and release as I spoke to Julian. I was terrified that Mark would somehow find out about my plan to leave him.

After talking to Julian about where I should go after I left Mark, I called our friends who lived up the coast to ask if I could possibly stay with them for a short while. It was a scary call to make, because somehow, it solidified my plan: I really was leaving.

I hadn't spoken to Tom and Rebecca in awhile, even though we had been close friends during college. They were one of the nicest couples I'd ever known; they started dating when they were in high school, continued through college, got married right after college, and they are still together today.

Like all my friendships, however, Mark had managed to drive a deep wedge in between us by trying to isolate me from everyone I knew, pressuring me to spend time only with him and his family. Although he had only a few friends, himself, he didn't allow me to get to know them at all. Most of them, I never even met. He would go play basketball with friends on Sunday mornings and have a barbecue at one of their homes afterward -- with their wives present and enjoying the day -- but he never invited me to join them.

When I called and told Rebecca what was going on in my marriage — sobbing my way through the description and, I'm sure, sounding only half coherent — she was immediately ready to help. She said that Sarah and I could stay there as long as we needed to, but I assured her it would be, at most, only a few days.

Then, I called my best friend, Kim. She was one of the few people I associated with somewhat regularly. We first met when I was in college and we didn't get along all that well. We lost touch shortly after I got married, and I always wondered how she was doing. One day, I was pushing the cart in the supermarket, with 6-week-old Sarah strapped to my chest, when, out of the blue, I heard Kim's voice: "Lucy, is that you?"

Our friendship was rekindled — or rather, "kindled," since we weren't good friends before — and we remain close to this day, 20 years later.

Kim is one of those people who has a deep understanding of human nature and, for better or worse, has learned a lot of life's hard lessons. Mark didn't like her and thought she was a bad influence on me because she was divorced.

I told Kim what I was planning to do, and why — and when. By this point, the countdown had begun and I only had about two days left. As strange as it sounds, I never thought of confiding anything to her about the state of my marriage, mostly because I didn't really understand the state of my marriage. My mind was so clouded, I could not even begin to articulate what was wrong. I just knew that my daughter was scared, and I had to leave.

Not wanting to create a panic with my parents and my family, I did not inform them beforehand and decided to wait until I was safely away to tell them what was going on. Instead, I told only Kim where I would be staying, and I planned to leave a note for Mark telling him just that. If he needed to reach me (God forbid), he could give a message to Kim, who could relay it to me.

So I had a place to go — a real escape route. But there was a lot left to consider before I walked, or ran, out the door. And I had to be so very careful not to show any sign of distress in front of Mark. He absolutely could not suspect that I was planning to leave him, or I might never get the chance.

SUITCASE

I remember the bay window in the bedroom, the light streaming in through the white shutters. It was warm and beautiful August weather in Los Angeles, as perfect as everyone imagines California to be.

My suitcase was on the floor underneath the bay window, right next to Mark's. We had started packing for our Mexican vacation several days earlier because it had been a busy time. His sister had gotten married, little Sarah was in the wedding, I was the pianist in the wedding — lots of things going on. On the surface, I looked normal, whatever normal looked like within this marriage. I played my part. I packed my suitcase for our vacation.

But underneath, nothing was normal. I had made my decision to leave Mark, and I only had a couple of days to get myself organized for my and Sarah's escape.

On top were my bathing suits and beach clothes. Underneath were some extra shoes and regular clothes, my personal papers, passport and Sarah's birth certificate. I also packed some extra clothes for Sarah in there, too. I remember wishing we had gotten her a passport, too, in case I wanted to leave the country. A mistake, but one I would have to live with.

I wanted to write a list of other things I needed, but I was too afraid Mark would find it. So I kept a mental list as best I could, considering the state of mind I was in.

I also was afraid Mark would rummage through the suitcase, but I took a chance and left it on the floor, right next to his.

MENTAL LIST

Here are some things I needed:

- Clothes and shoes to last both Sarah and me at least a week, maybe longer
- Toiletries for both of us
- My personal papers: birth certificate, passport, anything like that
- Papers related to Sarah, like her birth certificate and health records
- Things I didn't want Mark to destroy before I could retrieve them: Sarah's baby photo albums, a couple of my personal photo albums, gifts my mom had made for Sarah, Sarah's baby videos
- A few household goods, like things I might need to set up an apartment — but only if I took duplicates and only if they fit in the car; if not, they'd be left behind

- Some toys and books for Sarah
- Sarah's portable crib, sheets, blankets
- Sarah's stroller

Then there was money. We had a lot of cash stashed in the house, because many of Mark's clients paid him in cash and he didn't want to deposit it in the bank, where it could be traced (and he'd have to pay taxes on it). I thought I knew where all of it was hidden. Turns out, I didn't. I counted how much there was, in the one hiding place I knew of, and it came out to $10,000. I intended to take $5,000. I often wonder how much Mark had stashed in other places, like in the storage shed in the back yard where, a few weeks later, I went to retrieve some personal items and found two boxes torn apart, as if someone were frantically looking for something. Apparently, Mark found what he was looking for, because I never knew about that cash hiding place.

This is a fairly hefty list, and I had to keep it all in my head despite the mounting fear I was dealing with. And I also had to be able to grab all of it, pack it into the car, and drive away as quickly as possible after Mark left for work in the morning. I could not give him an opportunity to return and find me in the midst of my escape — which was a definite possibility, since he sometimes forgot something at home that he needed for work and would return within 20 or 30 minutes to retrieve it.

I also needed to scribble a note and leave it for him, all while making sure Sarah was OK. This was the best escape I could plan. So I braced myself for whatever was going to happen.

FEAR OF DYING

During the final days of my life as Mark's wife, my mind was in a frenzy.

I quickly made plans for where to go, what to bring with me, and when, exactly, to leave. I tried my best to keep calm in front of Sarah, who was only 2 years old at the time, and of course I told her nothing about what was going to happen.

But most of all, the fear of him finding out my plans nearly overwhelmed me.

During the day, when I wasn't on the phone with my friends to work out details of my escape, I was either trying to keep a sense of normalcy with Sarah or, if she was asleep or playing at a friend's house, crying hysterically and hyperventilating.

It was one of the times during my marriage to Mark that I literally thought I might die. I thought, Mark is going to see that I'm acting strangely, and he'll confront me and try to kill me.

Each day during that final week, as the clock would tick down toward the time Mark would open the door when he returned from work, I struggled to keep myself together. I swam in the pool to try and calm down. I scrubbed the house from top to bottom. Sarah and I went on walks or to the playground. Being with her helped, because it also put an exclamation point on my reason for leaving. But seeing her oblivious to what I was planning to do, and knowing the upheaval that was about to happen, nearly broke my heart in half.

The night before Mark and I were to leave on our trip to Mexico was actually the night before I was to leave him. By the time that night arrived, I just wanted it all to be over, like the feeling before you have surgery or get a tooth pulled. Just wake me up when it's over.

All I wanted was for Sarah and me, literally, to live through the next day.

THE NIGHT BEFORE

The night before I made my escape was, in actuality, rather fitting to the occasion.

Mark's sister Pam had gotten married, and she and her new husband decided they wanted to have a little party with the family while they opened their wedding gifts. Since parties usually seemed to happen at our house, Mark and I hosted it. We didn't make a huge fuss, but we did serve a nice meal, and everyone was there: Mark's parents, his other two sisters and one brother-in-law, two young nieces, perhaps a cousin or two.

We spent the evening oohing and aahing over the new couple's gifts. Mark and I also talked about our family vacation to Mexico, since we were scheduled to leave the next afternoon, after Mark did some work in the morning.

But I wasn't really there.

I made a good show, as I always did. I acted my part. I served the food, cleaned up any messes, took care of Sarah and made sure she had a good time, talked with the family.

All the while, I was reviewing my mental checklist over and over again. Money, papers, crib, photo albums. Toys, books, linens, clothes, baby videos. I envisioned Mark leaving for work in the morning, and then I pictured how I was going to gather everything together and put it in the car while also watching Sarah. I hoped she might actually sleep in a little late, so I could do the packing part without having to worry about her.

Then I imagined myself writing the note to Mark and leaving it on the dining room table: I have left with Sarah and am not coming back. If you need to reach me, please call Kim at this number. She is the only person who knows where I am.

When Mark's family left, I truly felt like I was saying a final good bye to them. In truth, it really was final. I never saw most of them again.

IT WAS A SUNNY DAY

August 31, 1990, was a beautiful sunny day. Not too warm, pleasant with a comforting breeze.

I barely slept the night before, anticipating what was to happen. The contrast between my fear and the warm sun was so sharp, it stung.

As usual, Mark got up early to go to work. He typically left by 7 a.m. or so. That particular day, we were scheduled to leave on a vacation to Mexico in the afternoon, but because he had clients to attend to, he decided to work until noon. I pretended that I wanted to finish packing for the trip, so I got up early, showered, and fussed with my suitcase.

Sarah woke up shortly before Mark left for work. I tried not to look rushed as I quickly got her out of her pajamas and into some clothes and set her up for breakfast. Small talk with Mark about the vacation, what time he'd be home so we could get to the airport ... my mind wasn't paying attention at all.

Did I fill up the car? Yes. How quickly can I get everything packed into the trunk? Maybe 15 minutes. What do I do if Mark comes back before I've left, if he's forgotten something?

That question, I had no answer to. All I did was pray that he wouldn't.

Around 7 am, I realized that Mark really had no idea what I was going to do. I had kept my secret, hidden my fears and anxieties. A few moments later, Mark walked out the door, started up his truck, and drove away. I listened to the engine noise fade into the distance, and then I started running: first, to the money.

I grabbed a footstool, climbed up to the highest bookshelf in our family room, and grabbed the entire wad of cash from our hiding place. I quickly counted to make sure it was $10,000, as I remembered. I counted out $5,000 and shoved it in my pocket.

Next, I grabbed the photo albums and baby videos from the bookcase and stacked them next to the front door. I ran to the filing cabinet in the back room and found all my personal paperwork, anything I thought Sarah and I might need.

I checked on Sarah, who was still eating her breakfast and not really paying attention to me.

On I went like this, running from one area of the house to the next, grabbing what I thought I needed: the packed suitcase, with my and Sarah's clothes hidden underneath our bathing suits. Toiletries, a few kids' books and toys, her favorite blankets my mother knitted for her, some tiny mementos.

Anything I could stuff into the car quickly, I took: A few linens, a few plates and silverware, even some canned food.

Then I opened the front door, ran to the car, which was parked in our carport, unlocked it and popped the trunk, and began to throw things in.

Back and forth I went, making several trips within a span of maybe 10 minutes. It all seemed to be taking just too goddamn long. And I still hadn't written the note or settled Sarah into the car.

Every time a car or truck would approach the house, my heart would stop for fear that it was Mark.

After about 20 minutes of running, I paused and decided that I had everything I could possibly take with me at that moment. I took a piece of scrap paper that we kept by the phone, scribbled the note to Mark, signed it, and left it sitting on the kitchen table, held down by an empty glass.

Sarah had finished eating, so I popped her into the bathroom for a 30-second wash-up, took one last look at everything, grabbed my purse, and bolted for the door.

I shut it behind me, locked it, and ran for the car, clutching Sarah close to me. I quickly belted her into her car seat, shut all the car doors and the trunk, got into the driver's seat, and slid the key into the ignition. I started the car.

Knowing I was possibly a dangerous driver at that moment, I allowed myself about 15 seconds of deep breathing before I put the car into reverse. The last thing I wanted was to have an accident.

I backed carefully out of the driveway, turned the car in the direction of the freeway, and stepped on the gas.

Mark's truck was nowhere in sight.

PART III

I THOUGHT IT WAS OVER

The moment I drove away from my house, away from Mark, I thought my nightmare of living in fear was over. I still didn't put a name to it, domestic violence. But I really believed that I was free, that Sarah was free, and that we would never be harmed by Mark again.

I remember driving on the freeway, nearing my safe haven, the home of my dear college friends Tom and Rebecca, and feeling high. I tore off my wedding ring and threw it into the glove compartment. I rolled down the front windows of the car, opened the sunroof as we approached the coastline, turned up the radio and started singing.

Sarah joined in — well, she didn't exactly sing along, but she "danced" in her car seat.

At that moment, I was happy. Truly happy. Scared out of my wits, yes. Afraid Mark would find us, yes. Psychologically damaged, of course.

But that could not outweigh my happiness at being out of that house. I thought it was over.

Sadly, it wasn't. Not at all. I wouldn't know that for many months, when my new life and new outlook came to a screeching halt.

For the moment, though, I envisioned that I had a real future. Life had more for me than what I had already experienced. After all, I was only 29 years old.

EMBARRASSMENT

It's tempting to underplay the embarrassment suffered by victims of domestic violence. Speaking solely for myself, it's still a problem for me, decades later. I have told very few people about what happened to me, and I've told even fewer about what happened to my daughter.

For me, the embarrassment stems from believing that I should have made different choices: I should have left after the first rape. I should have left after the second rape, or the third. I should have left after the first time he called me names, got in my face, threatened to kill me.

Intellectually, I know there were many reasons, good reasons, why I didn't leave before Aug. 31, 1990 — nearly seven years into the marriage. Mostly it was because I was trying to figure out the best way to stay alive.

Let me repeat that: I was trying to figure out the best way to stay alive. It's that serious. It really is.

But still, the embarrassment, the shame, lingers. I am

smart. I am educated. I had a lot going for me in my youth, including good looks (which are, sadly, fading now). Even at this moment, as I'm typing these words, the shame is welling up inside me, like a salty, bitter wave that I just don't want to taste anymore.

But here it is.

And here is another chapter by me, the writer using a pseudonym. Ashamed — yes, that is part of it — to reveal who I am.

Splintered.

Cracked.

Crumbled.

Mangled.

Ruptured.

Shattered.

Shredded.

A lot of synonyms for the same word: Broken.

I am still broken inside. There are parts of me that I can no longer find, although I keep searching because I can still feel them somewhere, somewhere: like an inner sense of lightness I used to possess, a high level of academic ability, and a strong sexual desire.

There are other parts of me that were simply obliterated the moment Mark first raped me, as though they were blown up by a bomb. It's difficult to explain the sense of fragmentation.

Parts of me became numb in order to protect my psyche from the violence, and those parts have eventually fallen away and died, like the ability to trust easily and my belief in a general kindness of people

Other parts of me — my self — retreated into hiding and still cannot be coaxed from the shadows.

And still other parts of me have remained, but have changed irrevocably. I may be stronger emotionally than I was before the abuse, but I've sacrificed some of my sensitivity and willingness to be vulnerable, for example.

This continually searching to find the pieces of myself is exhausting.

Should I quit? How could I possibly quit looking for my self among the rubble, as if stopping the search for a missing loved one whose body was never found?

IMMEDIATE AFTERMATH

*P*erhaps it's fortunate that I have only flashes of memory of the days immediately following my escape. When I arrived at my friends' home, far away from Mark, I left everything in the car except bare essentials for Sarah and me, so the car was still filled with all my stuff. I remember thinking, Is this really what my life is? A trunk full of linens, photo albums, and a suitcase?

Still very afraid that Mark would find us, I did not sleep well those first few days. I talked to Julian on the phone sometimes, and he helped me to think a little more clearly, at least for that moment. He was a good friend to me, as were the people with whom we were staying. They were truly generous with their time and help.

I remember one day, perhaps two days into my stay, when I found myself yelling at Sarah. Really screaming. I don't know what for, but clearly it wasn't because of anything she had done but simply because my stress level was sky high. My friends intervened and helped me to calm down as I collapsed onto the floor and cried until I couldn't cry anymore.

I also remember Sarah having a meltdown in a department store during that first week. Yes, she was 2 years old, and 2-year-olds have tantrums. But this was not a tantrum, I could tell. Even through my own emotional haze, I could see that she was completely stressed and just had to let it out — even if it was in the middle of a department store.

While I was at my friends' home, Mark apparently wasn't at our home. My friend Kim, who was the only other person who knew where I was staying, phoned me and said Mark had called and told her he was in Palm Springs for a few days.

I remember thinking, That's a bit odd. But maybe he'll leave us alone, if it's true.

What else was odd: Kim called me a couple of days later and asked if I knew a woman with red hair, perhaps a friend or client of Mark's. I knew all of Mark's clients, and he didn't have many friends. That description did not sound familiar. Kim said she saw the two of them together at a restaurant.

I was confused, until the first preliminary court appearance in early Sept., about a week after I filed for divorce and about 10 days after I moved out. There she was, the mystery woman, sitting with Mark in the courtroom.

News flash: Mark had been having an affair.

WHO IS SHE?

The mystery woman turned out to be named Lydia, a British nanny who worked at the home of one of Mark's biggest (and most famous) clients. I have no idea how long Mark had been seeing her while we were married. And of course, I started to wonder how many other affairs he had had while we were married. I think I can be pretty certain she wasn't the first.

When things started to come out during the divorce proceedings, facts about the abuse Mark inflicted on me, I thought, Certainly Lydia wouldn't want to stay with him once she learns about all of this. Who would take that kind of risk?

Apparently, Lydia did not believe any of it or was in denial. Because she did stay with Mark. They dated for four years and finally got married, and they're still married today.

When I think about all that has happened, Lydia is still the most confusing piece of the puzzle. I will never know what she really thought about everything back then, nor will I ever understand how she truly felt about Sarah. She was never Sarah's protector, even though she pretended to be her friend.

Even today, all these years later, I still ask myself this question about Lydia: Who is she?

A PHOTO OF THE REAL ME

*R*ecently on Facebook, my dear college friend Scott posted a photo that I remember very well. It's of a big group of us: Scott, Julian, Tom, Rebecca, Kim, me, and a couple more of our closest friends in college. It was either 1981 or 1982, but I think 1981, and we all look really happy and carefree.

And I look like me: the me I remember.

It's not just the blush of youth. I have a genuinely happy smile: glad to be alive, in love with life (and with Julian, at the time).

After what I've been pondering recently about being a broken person, the photo was a startling validation of what I believe to be true — about being fragmented, lost and, in some important ways, simply gone. The woman in that picture ceased to exist just a couple of years later. She may have been young, but she was no longer happy, no longer carefree, no longer glad to be alive much of the time.

I have found some happiness in my life since then. But only some.

Yes, I have my wonderful daughter. And yes, I eventually remarried, but it hasn't been an easy relationship, mostly because — I believe — I'm not a whole person. Many days, I feel simply like a shell: a female exterior with nothing inside. There are huge gaps in who I am vs. who I used to be, gaps that I have been unable to fill with any sort of "replacement parts." There's no such thing as spare parts when it comes to one's psyche.

I love looking at that picture of me, pre-domestic violence. It reminds me that I used to be really happy, and I'm grateful for that.

CREDIT CARD LESSON

About a week after I moved out, I had a major problem: the car broke down. Seriously broken down. The repair was covered under the warranty, but I was going to have to rent a car for at least a week.

I was very familiar with the folks at the dealership, as I brought the car there for all of the service appointments. They were very nice, and they always did a great job with the car. So of course, I took the car straight there for the repair.

When the nice man at the dealership explained that the repair would take a week or so, he also offered to help me with a car rental. Sometimes they had loaner cars available, he explained, but not for a week. I understood — no problem. So he got on the phone with the car rental agency they used and said they could start the process over the phone, and then bring the car to me. Since Sarah was with me at the time — she was just over 2 years old — I appreciated the convenience.

While he was on the phone, I handed him a credit card.

He gave the number to the rental agent on the other end of the line. Suddenly, he looked at me with a very strange expression. He said, very quietly, "I'm sorry, but this card has been canceled. By law, I can't hand it back to you. Do you have another one?"

He was so kind ... as we went through this process three more times.

Mark had canceled all of our credit cards, without bothering to tell me, of course. They were all in his name.

Except for one.

I realized that I had one credit card that was in my name only, from when I was in college. I never actually used the card, but it was valid, and it was in my wallet.

Important lesson: When you're married or in a relationship, always have at least one credit card that is only in your name.

SOLICITATION

Two weeks after I moved out of the house, I had to return there to get a few more of my things — just basics, not all my personal items.

I alerted Mark and his attorney of my visit, as required, and told them exactly what I was going to take from the house — nothing of value, just some clothes for myself and for Sarah, and a couple of toys. I tried to make it fast. I went into the bedroom with a small duffel bag and packed a few more clothes. I then went into Sarah's room and grabbed a few of her clothes and a couple of toys, just as I promised I would. Nothing more.

Before I left, I went into the kitchen to grab a glass of water. I was so nervous and scared, my throat had gone completely dry.

Mark came home.

He found me in the kitchen with the glass of water in one hand and the duffel in the other.

In that instant, I thought maybe he might try to kill me. We had seen each other only in court or with our attorneys by that point, not alone with each other.

But instead of trying to physically hurt me, he solicited me. That's right: he asked me if he could pay me to have sex with him.

He came very close to me, in an overtly sexual and provocative manner, and said, "I know you could use some extra money. I'll pay you to have sex with me. How much do you want?"

I was so stunned, I could barely speak. I almost thought he was kidding. Unbelievably, he wasn't. He asked me a second time, and I said — as calmly as I could, trying not to rile him — that I was not interested and had to leave.

Sometimes I still marvel that I escaped physically unharmed from that meeting. Maybe he was afraid that if he hurt me, it would harm his chances for a good divorce and custody agreement.

I felt so disgusted by what he said, a few minutes after I drove away I had to pull over. I thought I might vomit.

DOMESTIC VIOLENCE THERAPIST

For a short time after I left Mark, I saw a very good therapist who specialized in domestic violence. I'll call her Ann.

Ann was a kind and compassionate person who was extremely well versed in domestic violence. Part of her professional life consisted of counseling the abusers themselves (all men), so she had a good view of the situation from both a practical, realistic standpoint as well as from a researcher/professional one. And she saw both sides, too.

She told me that after all her years of working with the abusers (I'd guess she was in her mid-50s when I saw her), she had finally accepted the fact that men who engage in domestic violence against their spouses would almost never change. The rate of recidivism was nearly 100 percent. Only in rare cases did a man change his behavior, and it was only after having access to prolonged and intense therapy. And in this culture, that type of intense therapy is hard to come by due to insurance limitations and the like.

This news was very disheartening to me. When I first started seeing Ann, while I knew Mark and I would never reconcile, I had hoped we could have some sort of friendly relationship, for Sarah's sake. But after I moved out, his behavior became even more extreme.

For a while, in addition to private sessions I also attended small group-therapy sessions with other women who were victims of domestic violence. Many of them had experienced horrific crimes against them — two had been shot (one of them several times in the back, not sure how she survived), and one had been stabbed.

None of them, however, experienced two aspects of domestic violence that I had:

1. Sexual abuse/rape
2. Lack of a "honeymoon" period following a violent event, accompanied by an apology from the spouse

When I told the therapist and the other group members about those two facts, they stared at me in disbelief. They couldn't relate at all to the rape I described. I recall them saying, "My husband would never have forced me to have sex with him." This, from women whose husbands had shot or stabbed them!

Nor did they understand my point about my husband never apologizing for his actions. All of them said that after a violent event, their husband would later apologize, treat them well for a while, and buy them gifts or flowers.

Mark never did that. I have never, ever heard him say, "I'm sorry" — to anyone, about anything.

I continued in therapy, and Mark was going further out of control. At a certain point, Ann told me she couldn't help me anymore. What I was experiencing — after I moved out, mind you — was something she had never encountered, in all her years of working in domestic violence. I remember that she gave me a big hug and said she was so very sorry, but she did not understand this type of abuser — meaning Mark — and that she would refer me to some other professionals who could help.

One of them tried, with everything she had. I so appreciated her efforts. But she failed.

FLINCHING

~~~

After I left Mark, awhile later, I dated a police officer, named Don. Being a police officer, Don was very observant. Eventually, I told him about my marriage to Mark, and he was also someone in whom I confided what happened to my daughter. But I didn't tell him anything right away. It was a secret, and I felt ashamed.

The first time he suspected that I had been a victim of domestic violence was when he noticed me flinching. He would reach his hand out to me, to touch my shoulder or something, and I would flinch.

Of course, I didn't realize I was flinching. It had become a natural reaction to anything or anyone that came within a certain distance of my person.

At some point, Don asked me about it, about the flinching. I remember being afraid to tell him. I started to, and then I'd stop.

Don asked if I would be willing to watch a movie with

him, called "Sleeping with the Enemy." I realized later that, of course, he wanted to help me talk about what had happened to me, and he thought the movie would do that.

So we went to see it. I could barely watch it.

But it did help me talk to Don about my experience, although I did not tell him everything. How could I? I wasn't even at a point where I could be truthful with myself about my experience.

Seeing my reaction to the movie helped Don understand my flinching. And the movie may have helped me start to talk more about my experience. Therapy was helping, to a point — but only to a crucial point, and then it couldn't help anymore.

CONFUSION

During the first few months after I left Mark, my life was filled with confusion, swirling in circles without any clear direction.

I found myself a place to live, at least temporarily. It was far too expensive an apartment, but for the moment the court had forced Mark to pay me a decent amount each month — temporarily — pending the final divorce agreement.

The apartment building was on a busy street, but our unit was in the back so it was quiet. It had two bedrooms and one bathroom, no view except onto an alley. I knew we wouldn't stay there long, but it worked for a while. I filled it with rented furniture, except for a bed for me and a bed for Sarah, which I purchased. I wanted something of my own.

I had a new place to live, yes. But my heart and soul and mind were still lost, trying to find a connection to the new reality in which I lived. I felt a sense of freedom, but I still had to see Mark regularly to exchange Sarah for her visits. So I wasn't really free of him, and I still was frightened by him.

And I was dealing with the horrors of family law court (which is literally hell on earth — more on this later) and fighting against Mark, who thwarted me every chance he got in terms of a financial settlement. He still had power over me, monetary and emotional power.

I made some relationship mistakes in those first few months. I had a brief sexual fling with Julian, which nearly destroyed our friendship; I really was just using him to try and feel safe again, which did not work at all. We weren't ready, either of us, to have a relationship at that point. We didn't speak to each other for a very long time afterward.

I struck up the romance with the policeman. He was a nice man, but not right for me. Being with him, though, restored some of my self-confidence. I started to believe in my attractiveness again, and in large measure I have him to thank for that.

But being in any relationship at that point, just months after I left Mark, was clearly not something I could handle. My emotions ran hot and cold, and I had no sense of who I was as a person. How could I possibly bring anything of substance to a relationship?

All the while, I took care of Sarah and tried to make the rest of my life into something; I found temp work and also went to a post-bac program. I saw a domestic violence counselor who tried to help me. But I was so mixed up. I knew that at my core, I was damaged. The trauma inside me was palpable, like an inoperable tumor that could eventually kill my spirit, if not me. I felt as if I were freely breathing the air again, but at the same time I was standing on the edge of a cliff. My inner self was so wobbly, I really thought I might fall.

TRANQUILIZER

It is October of 1990. I am living in a temporary apartment with rented furniture, having moved out of my house Aug. 31, 1990. By law, once we started court proceedings, all of our money was put into a joint account and frozen, to be doled out by the attorneys as needed, and always notifying the other party first.

I call the bank to check on the amount in our account, because I need to pay my rent and buy some essentials.

The account, which had tens of thousands of dollars in it just a few days earlier, is now nearly empty. I almost faint.

I call my lawyer, who explains that Mark's lawyer indicated Mark needed the money to pay some business expenses. So my lawyer approved it.

I try to stay calm, explaining that half that money was mine, and now it's gone. I can't buy what I need to take care of my daughter or myself.

My lawyer says, "I'm sorry."

So now, I have no money. At all. Only what Mark has been ordered to pay me on a temporary basis, until we are able to reach an agreement on a permanent financial arrangement.

I call my doctor. For the first time in my life, I need a tranquilizer to calm down.

Incompetent, unscrupulous lawyers — I'm sure mine was on the take. His actions were so bizarre most of the time, he sometimes seemed like he was representing the other side.

$900

When the marriage dissolution was finalized — the custody part took much longer — I received $900 from my ex-husband. To live on. The judge ordered 3 monthly payments of $300, which he thought was enough in terms of time and money for me to find a job. I couldn't believe it.

When I moved out in Aug. of 1990, I had not worked in 2-1/2 years, because I had been on maternity leave and then had been staying home to raise our daughter (which we both agreed to).

When the temporary court order expired in early 1991, and then when the actual divorce was finalized in June of that year, I had almost nothing to my name. My ex had not been amenable to selling the house, in which he still lived, so he had to buy it from me — at a very, very reduced rate. He and his father also lied about a loan, saying we had not paid back his father (which we had). So that was deducted from the house sale.

I used nearly all of the proceeds to pay my attorneys' fees.

I lost everything, including my own piano (which my ex didn't even know how to play!). I had a pittance in the bank, enough to cover about one year of living expenses if I lived frugally. All I had left was the car and some – not all – of my personal belongings, many o which Mark destroyed before I could retrieve them from the house. My record collection, my books and family heirlooms – all of it was gone. Mark even got the house after buying my half at a rock-bottom price, He had refused to keep it looking good for potential buyers to see it, so we had no offers at all.

I received $900 in spousal support, total. For "family support," I received $700/month until Sarah turned 18.

To give this some context, in 1990 my ex-husband was making well into six figures per year, although he was only claiming about 40 percent of that on his tax returns. My lawyer and I tried to show how he was hiding money — he got paid in cash most of the time — but the judge would not listen.

The court system failed my daughter and me in ways that are unfathomable. I have often thought about writing a letter to that first judge, explaining to him what his decisions really cost us.

I have also thought about proposing legislation that demands a certain period of time for counseling if a woman has been the victim of domestic violence and is getting divorced. I made some terrible decisions because I simply wasn't thinking clearly. I filed for divorce just a few days after I moved out. Before I left Mark, I hadn't even thought about getting a lawyer first — definitely a mistake.

But then I remembered that the husband of one of the playgroup moms was a lawyer. Calling from my safe haven, I asked him if he would represent me, and he agreed. So one afternoon, I drove back to LA to sign the papers to file for divorce.

What I didn't realize that day was that in actuality, the family court system, at least in LA County, is seriously flawed. And I was in no emotional shape to navigate that system, and all its flaws, and make sound, rational decisions.

Unfortunately, my lawyers (I eventually had two from the same firm) didn't seem to understand that they were dealing with a traumatized victim of domestic violence. I needed a lot of help. But instead of pointing out the potential pitfalls along the way and helping me, they just went about their daily business and, in many cases, left me in terrible straits.

In total, during the 14-month court proceedings that ensued, I paid and/or lost upwards of $150,000 in the divorce settlement and lawyers' fees — fees that I paid monthly for years afterward.

When all was said and done, I had $20,000 in the bank and a 4-year-old car, plus lawyer bills and other bills to pay. Mark had a house worth several hundred thousand dollars plus everything in it, a new truck, a luxury leased car, plus any cash he'd hidden from me, which no doubt was considerable.

It's difficult to explain what it feels like to be denied what you believe are basic rights in a court of law. It's not exaggerating to say I felt like I'd been battered by the judge and the court system. It's also tough to fight against someone who lies, as Mark did in every single court appearance.

And as I was to learn, the legal system definitely favored Mark over Sarah. To the point where I almost decided to flee with her to Canada.

RECORD OF LIES, DESTROYED

For years, I had stashed all of the paperwork generated by all of our court proceedings in two brown, expandable folders. In there were all of the documents our lawyers submitted to the court, all the reports filed by psychiatrists/psychologists/therapists/doctors/police/social workers, all the correspondence — everything.

It was a huge pile of crap.

When I reached a point where I no longer had to keep any of it — which was just four years ago — I destroyed all of it.

Over the course of all those court proceedings, it became clear to me that, most of the time, the people in the court system don't care about finding the truth. They only care about getting people out of the courtroom as quickly as possible.

Literally every document Mark and his lawyer submitted to the court was a complete fabrication. Sometimes, I had no idea where on earth they came up with their ideas, they were so far away from reality.

Every time I looked through those documents — which I did a few times over the years — I almost got physically ill. It was difficult for me to believe that someone could just blatantly lie, over and over again, in what is supposed to be a court of law.

Mark did it in person, not just on paper. In one court appearance that had a huge effect on my financial situation after the divorce, he got on the witness stand and flat-out lied, saying that he and I had never agreed that I would stay home with Sarah after she was born.

By the time Sarah was born, Mark was making a lot of money. He never declared most of it on our tax returns, which I signed every year under extreme duress and threat of punishment. (I knew they were bogus.) But to provide some context, this was back in 1988. We were spending probably $5,000/month on whatever we felt like. That didn't even include our mortgage payment. And we still had tons of money left over to put in the bank.

And while I knew Mark hid cash around the house, I didn't know exactly how much. I found out later that he had several hiding places I never knew about. But at any given time, we probably had at least

$10-20,000 in cash hidden in the house. So there was no reason for me to work outside the home. And Mark and I agreed to that.

But he lied. The judge believed him, and he did not believe me: a sequence repeated over and over again.

All that paperwork only served to remind me that what appears in court documents is not the truth. The truth isn't even within a stone's throw. Anyone reading those documents would have no idea what our situation truly was, nor would they understand the cruelty that Mark inflicted on Sarah and me. The papers themselves were a form of abuse.

I felt like a weight had been lifted when I destroyed those papers with all those lies, as though a clearing had appeared in front of me and I could walk forward again.

BLESSING

*L*ong after I moved out and began to reflect on things that had happened, I realized that as sad as the miscarriage was, it also may have been a blessing.

First, of course, there may have been something wrong with the fetus. At least, that's what the doctor said. Not much consolation at the time, but it was all I had to believe in.

And if I had had a second child, I'm not sure I would have had the courage to leave Mark when I did. I might have stayed and continued to try to fix an impossibly broken situation. That was my nature then, and to some extent it still is my nature.

I understand why women who have multiple children stay with their abusers. It's a frightening prospect to be a single parent of one child, let alone more than one child. It's a tough life, especially if you aren't a millionaire (which I certainly wasn't).

I'm also glad that I did not bring a second child into the

relationship with Mark — yet another person for him to target with his violence. As much as I wanted a sibling for Sarah, it would not have been a good situation at all.

Unfortunately, I never had a second child. No sibling for Sarah.

But Sarah herself has been, and always will be, the biggest blessing in my life. Despite all she has endured during her life, she has maintained her beautiful, light spirit. Her eyes are wide open to possibility, and she enjoys life. She is strong, even stronger than I am.

LOST IN MY 20S ... AND MY 30S AND 40S

For my entire marriage and for many years afterward, I felt completely lost, without direction. I had no career path at all. I was intelligent, and I had a B.A., and I had a lot of skills. But I had no idea what to do with them. So I just found a job, any job, and worked. That was all.

At the time, I thought it was all my fault that I was so directionless. Now, I wonder how I managed to do as well as I did. I took a job as a legal secretary and stayed in that profession throughout my marriage. It was a demanding job, and I was good at it. I suppose it allowed me to escape my home life for a while and be focused on something else. I was fortunate that I worked for caring, nice lawyers who made my daily life interesting.

But it's difficult to make up for lost time. In my 30s, after my divorce, I tried to find a new career direction in writing and college-level teaching. I went back to school and earned two Master's degrees — took awhile to pay back the loans, but I did it. For many years, I split my time 50-50 between teaching and writing, though now I write full time.

Here I am now, at age 50, still sorting out what I really want to do with my career — and my *self*. I struggle every day to construct someone I recognize when I look in the mirror. Many days, I feel like a blank that's ready to be filled in, but with what, I just don't know.

It may be hard for people who have not been the victim of domestic violence to understand, but the truth is that as a result of being in this type of relationship, you doubt every aspect of yourself. It creates a mindset of, Can I trust myself? And that mindset permeates everything you do. Decision making, listening to oneself, moving in the direction of a career — it all becomes much more difficult.

JACKET

It was a cool day, sometime during the winter of 1990-1991. It isn't often that you had to wear a jacket or coat in LA, but this was one of those times.

By this point, I didn't have a ton of money to spend on clothes and things. Mark was still paying me a decent, albeit temporary, amount of money each month, ordered by the court so as to support me during the period before our divorce was finalized. But I was trying to be careful with money, especially since the lawyer bills were beginning to pile up.

It was a Sunday afternoon, and I was scheduled to go pick up Sarah from my old house, where Mark still lived. It was always awkward for me to return to the house, and I tried never to go inside when I picked her up there. If I saw Lydia, I usually said very little to her — she was basically living there by this point, just a few months after I moved out. And I also tried not to say much to Mark; it was just better that way. I still felt extremely nervous during these hand-offs and did not trust him to stay calm around me.

After all, I had embarrassed him by walking out on him. I walked out on him. Not a good thing to do to an abusive person who wants — needs — to be in control.

This particular Sunday, I remember being in a good mood because I had really missed Sarah that weekend and wanted to see her. I missed the energy of a 2-1/2 year old. I knocked on the door. She came running from inside the house and opened it, and Mark handed me her things. As usual, I quickly said good bye and turned to leave. Just when the door closed, I realized that Sarah had left her jacket inside — and she really needed it, as it was cold out. Even though it might have been simpler to forget about it, to be honest, I didn't want to buy a new one when she had a perfectly good one that she liked.

So I turned back to the house and knocked on the door again. The moment I rapped my knuckles on the door, I knew it was a mistake.

Mark didn't answer the door. Instead, he looked at me through the front window and mouthed, "What is it?" I replied that Sarah had forgotten her jacket, and could he please get it for me.

In an instant, he flew into a rage. I could hear him shouting obscenities, and he was literally running around the living room, waving his arms and turning red in the face. "Her JACKET? You want her fucking JACKET?" he screamed, over and over again. I picked up Sarah and turned to go, and suddenly Mark's fist hit the front window, right next to my face (and Sarah's). Thankfully, the glass didn't break.

Sarah cried out in shock, and we both rushed to the car to get away as quickly as possible. I realized, in that moment, that both of us were still in danger, and that much as I wanted to let them go, my feelings of fear with Mark were justified.

CHILD PSYCHOLOGIST

A few weeks after I left Mark, when Sarah and I were living in our first apartment, I noticed that she was exhibiting some signs of stress. She was irritable and her sleep was disturbed (she had always been a good sleeper), and she also was having potty accidents, which she hadn't had for several months.

It may seem obvious that she would be stressed, considering she had been uprooted from the life she knew, was living in a new place, and was going to stay at her old house sometimes with Mark.

She also had been introduced to Mark's girlfriend, Lydia.

I can only imagine how confusing all of this was to her, only being 2 years old.

But one specific thing really alarmed me, based on something my friend Kim said. Kim's young son and Sarah sometimes played together, so Kim had occasion to go to

Mark's house to pick up Sarah or drop off her son. What Kim told me one day was astounding.

In all respects, Sarah was — still is — a smart, well-behaved child. She liked books and quiet time, and while she really liked to be physically active and run around, too, she was rarely out of control. She was a typically vibrant 2-year-old, and she was a very easy child to parent because she actually listened and learned quickly what behavior was OK and what wasn't. I rarely had to issue any sort of punishment. It just didn't happen very often.

"She acts like an animal when she's at Mark's house," Kim said to me one day. "I don't even recognize her. She doesn't listen, she climbs all over everything in the house, she screams and yells. Honestly, she's like a completely different child when she's at Mark's house."

I had never, ever seen Sarah act like that. I hadn't worked outside the home since I gave birth to her, so I was with her every day of her life, up until the point she started going to Mark's house for visitation during our divorce proceedings. That her personality seemed to shift so drastically when she was there ... it concerned me.

Yes, she also was now in day care, because I had to do whatever temp work I could get to help with the bills. She had actually seemed to like being around other kids, and she made friends easily. But when she was with me, which was still most of the time, she did not behave "like an animal." She was her normal Sarah self, albeit slightly stressed.

So I took her to a child psychologist — and, as required by a temporary custody agreement, I told Mark I was going to do this. Dr. Smith, I'll call her, did a thorough check and determined that Sarah was under stress, but that she seemed very resilient and was going to be fine. She just needed time to adjust to the new living arrangements and to Lydia. I said I figured there was nothing to worry about, and I thanked her for her time.

We were both wrong. So very, very wrong.

PART IV

THE LIGHT WAS PINK

The light was pink as it came in through the windows. I had chosen rose-colored shades for Sarah's room in our second apartment, which was homier than the first place we lived. This apartment felt more like a little house, as it joined the apartment next door by only one wall and had a front and back door.

Although it was very noisy — on a busy street and also across from the freeway — it seemed like a home. I actually bought some furniture (instead of renting this time) and even bought a piano my brother wanted to sell.

As I put nearly 3-year-old Sarah to bed that night, on Memorial Day weekend of 1991 — 8 months after I left Mark, but before our divorce was final (we were still thrashing out the finances and custody arrangement) — I noticed how pretty the light looked as the sunset blended with the rosy hue of those shades.

I was looking at that beautiful light when my life changed. Forever.

As I knelt by the bed and began to say our prayers, Sarah was holding my right hand. Then something happened.

She started to lick my fingers. In an extremely provocative, non-toddler way.

It was literally as if I were thrown into an X-rated movie. The jolt to my whole system was so enormous, I felt as if I were going to faint.

I have no idea how I managed to do what I did next, but somehow all my strength — every ounce of courage and fortitude I possessed — kicked in.

I didn't pull my hand away. Instead, in a very calm and composed voice, I said, "Have you ever done that with anyone before?"

Sarah: "Uh-huh."

Me: "Really? Who?"

Sarah: "Daddy."

Me: "You lick Daddy's fingers like that?" I was still calm and composed, at least on the outside.

Sarah: "Yes."

Me: "Does Daddy lick you, too?"

Sarah: "Yes."

Me: "Where?"

Sarah grabbed her private parts. Me: "OK. Anywhere else?"

Sarah pointed toward her bottom.

Me: "I see. And do you lick Daddy anywhere else, other than his hands?"

Sarah: "Sometimes. On his bottom."

At that, she started to look a little distressed, so I decided to end the conversation. And I was desperately trying to stay calm and wasn't sure I could go any further without faltering.

Me: "OK. Thank you for telling me. Good night, sweetie pie."

I kissed her good night and went out into the living room. I collapsed on the hardwood floor, and my heart splintered.

I've rarely had the feeling that I literally had to pick myself up off the floor. But after Sarah revealed to me that her father had been sexually abusing her, that's exactly what I had to do.

After sobbing rather hysterically on the living room floor for about five minutes, I pulled myself together as much as I could, literally crawled to the sofa, and decided I needed to make a phone call.

I called Dr. Smith, the child psychologist who had seen Sarah several months earlier when I was concerned about her stress levels related to Mark's and my divorce.

Since this was after hours, I figured I would get her answering service, which I did. I provided my na

me, and in the message I said it was urgent because I suspected my daughter had been sexually abused by her father.

And Sarah was due to see Mark again in two days. I had to act fast. About two minutes after I hung up the phone, Dr. Smith called me back.

Dr. Smith: "Hello. I got your message."
Me: "Thank you for calling back so fast, Dr. Smith."
Dr. Smith: "Can you bring Sarah into the office?"
Me: "When?"

Dr. Smith: "Right now?"

I stopped for a moment and thought about the implications of that question, which were many.

Me: "I would do that, except she's asleep now."

Dr. Smith: "OK, I understand. Can you bring her in at 9 tomorrow morning?"

Me: "Yes, of course. I'll see you then."

Click went the phone, and my brain. This is about as serious as it gets, I thought, as I still gasped for air between sobs. What is going to happen?

That night, I made several other calls, all of which were emotionally charged. I called my family and my closest friends, including Tom and Rebecca, the people I stayed with when I moved out of the house.

When that particular friend answered the phone, I remember that for a moment all I could say was my name. When it was obvious that something was wrong and she asked me what had happened, all I could say, with a slight scream in my voice, was, "He molested her. He molested her."

That's the phrase that kept repeating in my head as I tried to go to sleep that night.

MANDATED REPORTER

*D*r. Smith, being a child psychologist in LA, was a mandated reporter. If she suspected abuse, she had to report it to the police, Child Protective Services, whomever else is on that particular list.

I took Sarah to see Dr. Smith the next morning, as planned. Dr. Smith asked Sarah several questions, which she answered as well as she could; she was just under 3 years old.

About 20 minutes into the session, Sarah became quite agitated and kept wanting to change the subject. And then, almost like flipping a switch, she stopped talking altogether, ran to the other side of the room, and curled up in the fetal position next to a giant stuffed bear.

I had never seen her do anything like that before. Never.

My shock must have registered openly on my face, because Dr. Smith turned to me and said, "I know this is very difficult for you to witness, and probably even to grasp, at this point. I have to tell you, however, that I do believe that your daughter has been sexually molested by her father, and I will need to contact the authorities."

THE AUTHORITIES

All I could think of at that moment was, The authorities will help me protect my child from this monster. I'm sure they will. That's what they're supposed to do. Everything will be OK, now that this is all out in the open. It will all be OK.

Such naiveté on my part. I had no idea what was ahead of us.

It's difficult to describe the depth of pain I felt, not just in the moment of Sarah's revealing what her father had done to her, but also in the hours, weeks, months and years afterward.

As a parent, your foremost responsibility is to keep your child safe. I didn't do that.

I know all the rational arguments to the contrary:

- You didn't hurt her. Her father did.
- You can't be responsible for something of which you have no knowledge.

- He hadn't shown any signs that would have led you to believe he would molest your daughter.

I could go on for days with these rational statements. I understand all of this, in my head. To this day, my heart cannot fully accept it.

She is my child. And my child was hurt, by someone who I knew was capable of violence. No, I never pictured him as being capable of — or even thinking of — molesting our daughter. Not being a violent, abusive person myself, these things don't readily come to my mind (thank God).

Even knowing all of that, I still hold myself responsible to some degree. I should have recognized some signs. No, there were no physical signs of this abuse. As a social worker told me, "These people are clever. They know how to do things that won't show up on a physical exam."

I chalked up Sarah's slight behavior changes — sleep disturbances, potty accidents, for example — to the stress of going through the divorce process and also having to make friends with a new woman in Mark's life. So much change, in such a short time, must have been frightening for a 2-year-old girl.

I never imagined, though I can see it clearly now, that some of those signs were related to the abuse she was suffering. Her out-of-control behavior at Mark's house seems like a way to try and cope with the pain of what was happening to her. She had to let it out somehow.

What else bothered me was that I had no idea how long

the abuse had been going on. I have to believe it was already happening while I was still living with Mark.

My mind went in a million directions as I tried to sort out how this could have happened, and more to the point: why? I still ask the question, Why would a father do this to his own child?

CHILDREN'S HOSPITAL

After I took her to see Dr. Smith, I was required to take Sarah to Children's Hospital for an "official" physical exam. I believe it was later the same day, although my memory is a bit fuzzy on that.

Suffice it to say, this was a troubling thing to have to do, to bring my daughter, not even 3 years old, to a hospital for a physical exam regarding sexual molestation.

I was allowed to be in the room with her for the exam, but I was not allowed to be very close to her. I couldn't hold her hand, and I couldn't talk to her. I was close enough for her to see me, and the doctor who did the exam was very kind and, thankfully, completed the exam as quickly as possible.

Of course, I couldn't really explain to Sarah exactly why we had to do all of this. Being a bright child, I'm actually quite sure she pieced it together somehow, in a way that she, at her young age, could grasp.

After Sarah had been examined and we were waiting to

hear what came next in this process, a social worker — I'll call him Greg — came over to talk to me.

Greg was a young man, about the same age I was, 29. He was a tad rotund, with friendly brown eyes behind oval spectacles. He told me he had read through the intake report and physical exam, and that he wanted to tell me something.

Greg: "I know this must be very frightening for you and your daughter."

Me: "Yes, it is. I'm trying to understand what's happened, and how it happened, and what's going to happen now."

Greg: "Listen to me now. I want you to understand something. These people, people who molest children, are extremely clever. They know how to abuse a child in a way that doesn't leave any physical evidence.

But just because there isn't any physical evidence doesn't mean that something didn't happen. I've seen this many times before, unfortunately."

My mind froze for a moment.

Greg continued: "Let me say this again: Just because there is no physical evidence of a crime, that doesn't mean a crime hasn't been committed. Always remember that."

I started to hear what Greg was telling me. Mark might actually get away with it. Greg is trying to warn me.

That's impossible, I corrected myself during my momentary interior dialogue. Surely with what Sarah has said, and some corroboration from a child psychologist, and further interviews that are bound to happen … she'll be safe now. Won't she?

The exam found had no physical evidence of molestation.

On the one hand, I was relieved; the thought of any physical harm being done was too horrible to contemplate. On the other hand, I still knew the truth: Mark had molested our daughter. Even if a physical exam won't support it, Sarah had told the truth. The psychologist believed her. The social worker Greg believed her.

And I believed her. There was no doubt in my mind as to what had happened, but I just wasn't sure the extent of it.

Why wouldn't people do everything in their power to protect her now?

RUNNING

The day after Sarah told me what had happened, the same day I saw Dr. Smith and, I believe, the same day we went to Children's Hospital, I was also in contact with my lawyers (I had two, by this point).

I was very worried because Sarah was supposed to go back to Mark for a visit the very next day. And I wasn't about to let that happen. I explained everything that had happened so far, with the psychologist and then at Children's Hospital, and I asked them what I should do.

My lawyers told me that they would be in touch with the authorities and the court and explain that Mark's abusive behavior has left their client (me and Sarah) no choice but to go away for a few days. We would return as needed to speak to the police and other authorities, but for a short time we simply had to go somewhere safe.

Major reality check.

It hit me like a brick: Mark is going to learn of this

accusation within a matter of hours. What is he going to do when he finds out?

That fear of being killed surged through my body, and I started to shake. I had to get myself together, because there was simply no time to waste.

I ran around the apartment and packed a few things, called around and found a hotel in which to stay, and called my family to ask anyone who could, to please come to LA and help Sarah and me. I told no one else where I was going except my family and my lawyers. Not even any friends this time.

Escaping. Running. Again.

MY MOTHER

$\mathcal{I}$ need to pause here and write about my mother. She deserves so much more than these few words, but for now ...

One of the last times I saw my mother healthy was when she and my dad joined Sarah and me at the hotel where we stayed for a week, on advice of my lawyers, after Sarah revealed her father had been molesting her.

I remember my mom and me, with Sarah taking a nap nearby, watching "Total Recall" in the hotel room and laughing at the goings-on of Arnold Schwarzenegger. She thought the whole thing was pretty funny, and we had a few laughs amid the awfulness that was going on in our real lives.

In July of 1991, about six weeks after Sarah's revelation, my parents, my sister and her husband (who had come to visit and see how we were all coping), Sarah and I went to Disneyland. We really needed a break, a day just to feel happy.

At Disneyland, my mother, age 71 and up until then super

healthy, began to have trouble keeping up, which wasn't like her at all. She was usually the one setting the pace for the rest of us (she walked faster than I did). But that day, she kept asking to sit down, and she skipped a lot of the rides.

A couple of weeks later, after she and my dad had gone back home, my mother got out of the pool — she swam every day at their condo complex — and could not catch her breath. My father was away, so she called my sister-in-law, who is a nurse. When my sister-in-law arrived, my mother was in dire straits and needed an ambulance. She was rushed to the ER and almost died. Her lungs were filled with fluid, and the doctors could not find the cause.

She recovered from that episode and started to get better. A few months later, in October, she had a major relapse and nearly died again.

(An aside: During this episode, her doctor called me, personally, in L.A. and said I needed to come to the hospital — in the Bay area — right away because she wasn't going to live more than a day or two, in his opinion. I was supposed to be in court the next day, so I called my lawyer and told him they were going to have to delay the appearance — I needed to see my mother, who was gravely ill. Mark's lawyer insisted that I get a signed note from the doctor literally — literally — saying that he believed my mother was going to die at any moment. So when I got to the hospital, that's what I had to do: ask the doctor for a goddamn note to "excuse" my court appearance.)

This time, the doctors found the cancer that had invaded my mother; small tumors, like blisters, were surrounding her heart and causing it to be constricted and also filling her lungs with fluid. The doctors never found the cancer's origin. She survived this particular episode, but she didn't have much longer to live.

She and my father opted to have her undergo chemotherapy, which lasted about four months. The treatments were stopped in March of 1992, and she died May 30, 1992, at age 72. I was 30 years old; Sarah was just under 4 years old.

To say that her illness and death added grief and stress to an already impossible situation — trying to finalize my divorce, dealing with the horrors of my child being sexually molested by her father and going through that legal process, while also attempting to recuperate from my own trauma — well, there really are no words.

Even though I was dealing with so much, I tried as best I could to focus on my mother when I was with her, which was nearly every weekend. I was either flying or driving there to see her, usually with Sarah along.

I was with my mother when she died. The next day, I flew back to L.A. to take care of some pressing legal business. On the return trip for the funeral a couple of days later, Sarah looked out the window of the plane and asked me, "Mommy, is this what the world looks like when we die?"

MORE AUTHORITIES

※

During the first few days after Sarah's telling me about what her father had done to her, we were in hiding from Mark but also having to deal with the authorities.

We were interviewed by the police, where Sarah was questioned about what had happened and also was "tested" about whether she knew the truth from a lie. For example, the officer would give her a crayon of a certain color, like purple, and then would ask her to give her the red crayon. Sarah responded, "But this crayon is purple, and that's not what you want."

The officer would say something like, "But you could give it to me anyway, right?" And Sarah would say, "But you asked for a red one."

The officer concluded that Sarah, age just under 3, knew the difference between the truth and a lie.

The officer, a woman, pulled me aside after the interview and said something that reminded me so much of Greg, the social worker at Children's Hospital, that it sounded like a recording.

Officer: "It's clear to me that your daughter knows the difference between the truth and a lie. However, there is no physical evidence to support her assertions about her father. Without that, I doubt that the DA is going to prosecute him. But remember this: Just because there is no evidence of a crime, doesn't mean that a crime hasn't been committed. Do you understand what I'm saying?"

Me: "Yes, I think I do."

I certainly did understand. And my fear was mounting. The authorities weren't going to be able to protect Sarah, I could see that now. I just didn't want to believe it.

FLOWERS AND SCREENS

About three days after Sarah and I went to stay at the hotel, we had to return to our apartment to meet with a different social worker, this one from Child Protective Services. He needed to see where we lived and how we lived, and how Sarah and I interacted at home.

I was very nervous about going back to the apartment, because I really feared how Mark must have reacted when he learned of Sarah's assertions. I thought perhaps he had trashed the place, or was lying in wait for us. Having lived with him for so many years, I knew what his anger looked like. Although I never dreamed he would molest our daughter, I certainly understood his temper and how much he needed to control people.

This accusation, coupled with the fact that I left him, must have made him feel more vulnerable than ever before. It truly terrified me, what he might do.

My parents drove with us to the apartment. A few weeks

earlier, I had taken the time to buy some flowers to plant all around the outside. Since the apartment shared only one wall, three sides were like a small house, with planters all around. So I had planted some petunias and impatiens to brighten up the place — they looked really nice.

That is, until I returned to the apartment that day.

Every single flower was torn out of the ground and tossed onto the grass.

Worse still, it was clear that someone had tried to break into the apartment. Every single screen (and there were many of them, probably about 10) was slightly pried open, but only bent — the person hadn't succeeded in breaking in.

Of course, we knew who had done it. I asked my next-door neighbors if they had seen anything, and they said no, that they'd only found the damage this morning and didn't know where I was.

Even though I did not want to feel afraid, I did. In looking at the damage, I knew it was done with pure anger and hatred, with Mark showing me that he was trying to find me and hurt me, and possibly Sarah, too.

Without proof or fingerprints (there were none), and with no real property damage done, I couldn't get anywhere legally. It was, however, a solemn reminder of how serious things were — as if I needed one.

THE QUESTION

I knew, right from the start, that Sarah was telling the truth. Many of the authorities we spoke to believed her too, even though it was becoming clear that they probably could do nothing to help us.

There was another reason that I believed Sarah, though. Mark never asked *the question*.

Mark never said, "I didn't do this to Sarah. And if I didn't do this to her, who did? And is she going to be all right?"

If he were a caring, loving father who hadn't hurt her but believed that something had happened, wouldn't he have asked that question? Wouldn't he have asked if she was OK?

He did not. He never even hinted that he was concerned about her. Instead, he went on the defensive, thinking only about himself. Denial, accusations about me and about Sarah. Not a surprise, perhaps, but distressing nonetheless.

I knew the truth. As difficult, almost impossible as it was

to accept, I knew what Sarah had said was true. No matter what Mark said or did, it did not change the reality of what he had done.

I just could not let him do it again. I had to find a way to keep her safe.

REPRIMAND

⁂

A week or so into this process, Mark and I had to appear in court. Obviously since Sarah had told me what had happened, the court needed to change the visitation arrangements pending the outcome of the whole investigation.

I asked the court to strip Mark of all visitation privileges while the investigation went on. The judge allowed visitation to continue.

I asked the court to assign an impartial monitor during Sarah's visits with Mark, in that case — someone the court could recommend who wasn't associated with us or the case in any way.

The judge denied my request. Instead, he assigned Mark's mother as the monitor.

So while this investigation took place, which also included an extensive evaluation by a court-appointed psychiatrist (of all three of us), Mark would still be allowed to see Sarah on the same schedule as before: every other weekend, and every Wed. evening.

The only changes were 1) Mark's mother had to be present, and 2) Sarah could not stay overnight. And I — yes, me — received a stern reprimand from the judge.

What did I do wrong, you may ask?

The judge admonished me for not informing Mark before I took Sarah to see Dr. Smith this time. He said I had broken the rules of our temporary custody arrangement by taking our child to see a psychologist without Mark's approval.

Yes, I was supposed to tell the molester of my child that I was going to take her to a psychologist to verify that, in fact, he had molested her.

The outright absurdity of that reprimand, coupled with the horror of the whole situation and knowing that Sarah was going to have to see Mark regularly again, really sent me into a state of anxiety.

I was starting to tumble downhill, into an emotional abyss that seemed to have no end. At every turn, it seemed, the authorities were doing everything they could to help Mark and not Sarah (or me, for that matter).

After being away for a week in the hotel, Sarah and I moved back into our apartment, and I tried — while continuing to deal with the molestation investigation — to resume living whatever kind of "normal" life I could, at that point.

For example, I gave myself a party when I turned 30, which also coincided with my divorce being finalized and my finishing an intense post-bac program at UCLA. I also tried to get out with friends as much as I could.

But I lost a lot of weight (which I couldn't afford to), I started having other health problems, and I couldn't focus on work. I was still temping and then took a permanent job, which I left after just a short time because, of all things, I found out the company was doing something illegal.

One thing in my life kept happening over and over again, something I could not stop: Every time I handed Sarah over to Mark, even though his mother was supposed to be present with them, I felt like I was literally giving her to the devil, to do with as he pleased.

There really are no words to describe how that feels.

And yet, I was the one the court reprimanded. I was told I could face jail time if I did something like that again.

I could face jail time. I thought, Well, if I'm at risk of facing jail time for that, I might as well take a real risk.

CANADA OR MEXICO

At some point during this whole nightmare, I considered chucking everything and taking Sarah to Canada or Mexico.

Unfortunately, she did not have a passport. If she had had one, I would have taken her to France and set up a new life for us there. I speak the language well enough, and I know their laws about extradition are fairly strict. I could not get her a passport without Mark's knowledge, so that was out of the question.

As it was, Canada and Mexico were my only options; neither required passports for entry at that time. Of the two, Canada seemed like the better choice because there would be no language barrier, jobs prospects seemed more likely, and the country has a good health care system.

In the end, though, I chose to stay in the U.S.

Why? I was idealistic. Despite everything, I thought that

"the system" would help me protect my child from harm. I needed to give it a chance to work, even though my fears were mounting that it wouldn't.

COURT-APPOINTED PSYCHIATRIST

❧

As the investigation into Sarah's allegations continued, the three of us — separately — saw a court-appointed psychiatrist.

Dr. Brown, I'll call him, was supposed to interview each of us and give us some psychological tests. Here's what it turned out to be, at least from my perspective:

1. A 5-minute conversation with Sarah
2. A 10-minute conversation with me, and a conversation with Mark of unknown duration.
3. An MMPI test for me and one for Mark, which I later discovered was scored incorrectly for me.

Apparently there are different ways to score the test depending on the person's psychological history. Mine was scored as if I had never been exposed to domestic violence or rape and did not have post-traumatic stress disorder, or PTSD.

The results of the MMPI tests showed me as a person who had trouble with intimacy, had (I'm paraphrasing) sexual hang-ups, was fearful and sometimes overreacted to potential danger.

All I could say to that was, DUH. But when I found out that the wrong scorecard had been used, it was too late to fix it.

The results of Mark's MMPI on the whole showed him as — seriously — more "normal" than I was. It noted that he had some mild problems with his temper that a couple of anger-management classes might help to correct.

And here is exactly how the psychiatrist's conversation with me started:

Dr. Brown: "You said your daughter described and demonstrated how her father sexually abuses her. Is that correct?"

Me: "Yes."

Dr. Brown: "Do you want it to be true?"

Me: "What? I don't understand your question."

Dr. Brown: "Do you want it to be true, that Mark sexually molested Sarah?"

I couldn't believe he was asking me that!

Me: "Of course I don't want it to be true. I don't want my daughter to have been sexually molested, by her father or by anyone else!"

I knew at that moment that there was something deeply

flawed about this whole process. Boy, was I ever right about that. It only went downhill from there.

DEPOSITIONS AND COURT APPEARANCES

The process of investigation led to depositions and court appearances. Dr. Smith, the child psychologist, appeared before the court and explained what she saw in Sarah that led her to believe that the molestation did, in fact, happen. Dr. Brown was also asked to report his findings in front of the court, as were a couple of other authorities.

Many of my memories of the court appearances are lost. It was such a painful, difficult experience that I believe my mind has blocked it from me.

What I do remember very distinctly, however, was the reaction of Mark's family and my family to the whole situation.

Whenever we appeared in court, my family was with me. They supported Sarah 100 percent and believed her completely.

Mark's family, including Lydia, his new live-in girlfriend,

supported Mark. NO ONE on his side of the family contacted me and asked how Sarah was doing. All this time, of course, Mark was still allowed to see Sarah during regular visitation sessions, as long as his mother was in the room. I have no way of knowing if they actually followed through on that provision, but I had no choice but to allow the visits to happen. Otherwise, I could have been sanctioned by the court or even sent to jail for disregarding a court order.

Also during this process, I was deposed, with my lawyers, Mark and Mark's lawyer in the room (along with a court reporter).

In one particularly brutal session, I had to describe exactly what Sarah had told me had happened. Mark looked me straight in the eye as I spoke.

While I was talking, I was pretty choked up. And Mark laughed. And laughed some more.

THE RULING

After about five months of slogging through this process, we got a ruling.

Beforehand, I had agreed in writing, on the advice of my lawyers, to abide by whatever Dr. Brown, the court-appointed psychiatrist, determined. My lawyers believed that by doing so, I was showing as much objectivity in the situation as I possibly could, and the court/judge would look favorably on that.

So here it was: The judge stated that Dr. Brown could not determine with certainty if any molestation had occurred. However, he did NOT believe that the mother (me) was lying or making up a story.

I have yet to understand how those two statements can be reconciled.

If I wasn't lying about what Sarah had said to me, then why wouldn't he know "with certainty" that she had been molested by her father?

The judge then ordered that we share legal custody 50-50 (meaning all major decisions had to be agreed to by both of us), and that Mark receive "liberal visitation" with his daughter, without a monitor present. I would be named the "primary custodial parent."

We were then asked to go into a room and hash out the details of the visitation arrangement and sign the paperwork.

I could not believe what I was hearing. And yet, I could. Many of the people I had met along the way had warned me that this would probably be the outcome. Their words reverberated in my mind: "Just because there's no physical evidence of a crime doesn't mean it didn't occur."

But when this ruling was finally handed down, it seemed impossible. What was I going to do now? How could I possibly abide by this agreement?

After the judge announced the psychiatrist's findings and recommendations, Mark and I and our attorneys went into a room to finalize everything on paper.

Mark ended up with the following:

1. Every other weekend, beginning Friday evening and ending Monday morning
2. Every Wed. night, overnight

He also got several weeks of sustained visitation during the summer, and holidays every other year. I protested. Loudly.

My lawyers told me there was nothing they or I could do to change the situation.

As I signed the papers, I announced to the court clerk that

I wanted it noted in the record that I was signing this agreement under extreme duress and pressure from both Mark and his lawyer and my own lawyers.

Thus began my new nightmare: leaving my beautiful daughter in the hands of her molester several times a month.

WHAT NOW?

My parents, the rest of my family, my friends and I couldn't accept the outcome of this whole court process. We simply couldn't understand how a child could be placed back into the hands of her abuser this way.

I kept wondering how it might have been different if she had revealed all of this about a stranger or a friend instead of her father. Would the authorities have been more likely to act on the word of a child, in that case?

By this time, which was late fall of 1991, my mother was quite ill and unable to travel. So my father came to LA to go along with me to meet with some potential new lawyers. I had to find out if there was any other legal recourse open to me. We kept asking ourselves, What now? What can we do now?

My father and I went to meetings with four other lawyers who specialized in child custody cases, all of them highly recommended.

At every meeting, the lawyers told us almost verbatim the same thing: This custody fight will cost you tens of thousands of dollars. And it won't work.

I suppose I have to commend them for telling us the truth and not just going after some money. But our truth was that we did not have tens of thousands of dollars. I had nothing left by this point, and in fact was going into debt just to survive. My parents had had some serious financial difficulties and were not in a position to help.

The "problem" was Sarah's age, the lawyers said. She was, as they put it, "too young to be believed without physical evidence to support what she's saying."

When I first started the divorce process, long before Sarah's statements, I discovered that in LA, the family court system is all about "reunification." (Ironic for divorce court, right?) In other words, they want children to have some sense of normalcy despite the parents being divorced.

I appreciate the sentiment, but it doesn't usually work. It certainly was not going to work for us.

And in our case, the court dismissed my statements about domestic violence and rape and Sarah's statements about her sexual abuse because, as they put it, "there is no physical evidence to support these claims."

Without physical proof, Mark's word — that he had done nothing — was gold. His statements were accepted by the court as fact.

Sarah's and mine — that he was dangerous and abusive — meant nothing. If the court had given any weight to what the two of us were saying, the judge's ruling would have been completely different.

The accused got the benefit of everything the court system could do. Mark got liberal visitation with his daughter, only had to pay me a total of $900 in alimony, got the house and everything in it, the cash that he hid from me, and on and on. He did not even have any lawyer bills; he paid his lawyer "in kind" by taking him on as a client.

The victims, Sarah and me, got nothing. And worse than nothing, Sarah had to visit her abusive father regularly, without me there to protect her.

Financially, we ended up with $700/month in child support and a stack of lawyer bills. I had about $25,000 in the bank on which to try and live until I could find a job, which wasn't going to be anytime soon because I needed to spend time with my mother, who was not going to live much longer.

My answer to the question "What now?" was becoming much more murky.

LYDIA

All through the custody hearings and the investigation into Sarah's molestation by her father, Lydia stood by Mark and supported him. She sat next to him in court, and she lived in his house.

What on earth was she doing?

At the time, I thought perhaps she was being abused by him, too, so she was going along to get along, as they say. Afraid to go against him, she decided to support him. That seemed relatively logical, considering what type of person is was/is.

I also thought maybe Mark had convinced her that I was lying. Knowing how persuasive and manipulative he could be, that, too, seemed like a logical conclusion.

Still, wouldn't she have had some doubts? Especially if she read or listened to my statements about the abuse I endured in combination with Sarah's description of what he did to her?

For the life of me, I could not understand what was going on.

Even though parts of the truth were revealed to me several years later, Lydia remains a mystery. Not everything adds up, and I guess I have to accept that it never will. This woman who became a central figure in my child's life will always represent a huge question mark, both to me and to Sarah. I think about her sometimes, and I wonder if she ever thinks about us.

NAIVE, BUT VIGILANT

In the months that followed the court ruling, which was that Sarah had to continue to see her father as before, despite her assertions that he had molested her, I remained vigilant. I watched for any and all signs that Mark was continuing to hurt her, and I tried my best to be calm whenever I had to hand her over to him.

To make things more sane, when I would arrive at the house to pick her up or drop her off I would try to find something positive about the situation, like having Sarah show me a new toy or playing with one of the pets. She loved a special cat there, named Sam. I came to understand much later how much Sam meant to her.

Mark and Lydia seemed — seemed — to be working on being more civil toward me. They would never invite me in the house for very long, but there were no more violent outbursts toward me. Whenever I showed up, things looked relatively OK; the house was not as clean as when I lived there, but it was fine.

I was very naive. Since I had learned from other attorneys that trying to fight the judgment would be fruitless, I convinced myself that Mark wouldn't continue to molest Sarah because he knew everyone was watching him. He wouldn't want to get caught a second time.

That was wishful thinking on my part. But what choice did the court leave me? My only other option was to flee the country with Sarah, but for obvious reasons that was not so easy — especially because I was essentially broke due to all the legal bills.

So I remained as vigilant as possible while I made plans to change the aspects of our lives over which I had control.

EASTER 1992

Over Easter of 1992, Mark and Lydia took Sarah on a vacation to Lake Tahoe, I think it was — someplace in the mountains, a reasonable driving distance away. I was extremely apprehensive about this trip, for a few reasons.

It would be the first time Sarah had really been far, far away from me since I moved out of the house in August of 1990.

I also remembered what Mark was like on vacation. His behavior was always at its worst, its absolute worst. For example, we were on vacation when he nearly strangled me, when Sarah was just a few months old and sleeping in a crib.

And of course, the thought of her being alone with Mark always made me anxious.

They were gone for three days, as I recall. And they were supposed to return in the early afternoon. They did not. These were the days before cell phones, so I had no way of reaching them.

An hour went by. No call from them. Two hours. Three hours. Four hours. Five hours late, and still no call.

As the afternoon turned to evening, and the evening turned to night, I became a little frantic. Since no one on Mark's side of the family was speaking to me anymore, I couldn't call anyone and ask if they had heard from them.

My anxiety began to turn into panic: What if he had taken Sarah, for good? What if he didn't intend to bring her back?

I tried to sleep but kept waking up. When the sun hit me in the face, I woke up with a start the next morning, realizing the phone had not rung all night. I busied myself as best I could around the apartment, my anxiety at a fever pitch.

Finally, at about noon, Mark pulled up in the car with Sarah. Lydia wasn't in the car, which meant they had stopped at home first. When I asked why he didn't call to tell me they were going to be almost a full day late, Mark said that the weather was so nice they just decided to stay and didn't think it would be any big deal.

It was a big deal.

As I came to find out later, these vacations that Sarah took with Mark and Lydia were a very big deal.

But I was just glad to have Sarah home with me. She was dirty and unkempt, but I didn't notice anything out of the ordinary about her behavior. I think, looking back, that she was already learning how to conceal what was really going on.

LA RIOTS, MAJOR DECISION

At the end of April 1992, the LA riots took over the city. By that point, I had lived in LA for 13 years, and despite my horrific marriage, I had enjoyed living in the city very much. It had always been an escape for me. I could drive to the beach, see beautiful homes, go shopping in fabulous stores, eat great food, and enjoy the gorgeous weather and do sports, like tennis and swimming.

That whole feeling was destroyed during the riots. I couldn't believe that the city I loved — the city I trusted — could turn upon itself in this way.

I remember vividly how that evening began. We all knew the King verdict was going to be handed down. When I heard the verdict, I was devastated.

My then-boyfriend, the police officer Don, and I were at my apartment watching the Lakers on TV. They were having a great game, and we were cheering loudly — trying not to think too much about the King case. (Incidentally, he was an expert in the baton and taught classes in using it, and he thought it was open-and-shut against the officers.)

Suddenly, my wonderful next-door neighbor came knocking on the door. I thought maybe we were being too loud, although he was a Laker fan and surely was watching the game, too.

"Have you seen what's happening?" he asked, his eyes wide. "Sure!" I answered. "The Lakers are having the best game ever!" "No! NO!" he shouted. "Riots are starting! Riots are starting!"

My police officer boyfriend reached for his pager and realized he'd left it at home. "I gotta go, right now," he said. "I'll try to call."

I didn't hear from him, nor could I reach him, for nearly five days.

One of my sharpest memories of that time was the curfew. As I've mentioned, Sarah and I lived in an apartment on a very busy street, right across from the freeway. It was extremely noisy at all hours; the freeway really never let up.

During the riots, the police/officials imposed a curfew: no one could drive from dusk until dawn. Suddenly, it was silent outside.

Deadly silent.

While the riots were happening, Sarah was at Mark's house, which made me all the more nervous. I wanted her with me, so she wouldn't be afraid.

And on top of that, my family had already planned to take my mother, who was gravely ill, on one last trip to my sister's cabin in the Sierra Nevada. The trip was to begin on what turned out to be the second day of the riots. Even though I was afraid to leave Sarah behind in the turmoil, I drove the long, long way to the cabin to spend some time with my family and my dying mother.

Although we focused on her, we naturally followed what was happening in LA, too. That brief trip was an emotional rollercoaster for me. One minute, I was talking to my mother about how she wanted her funeral, and the next minute I was watching TV trying to figure out if my neighborhood was under siege and if my then-boyfriend was OK.

After two days in the mountains with my mother, I drove back to LA; the riots went on for another three days. (The policeman was unhurt but traumatized by what he had seen.)

People were injured, many of them. One of the most severely injured, Reginald Denny, was the father of one of Sarah's friends at her preschool. That really hit close to home.

And people died.

Buildings went up in flames.

Although the major looting and violence had stopped, when I drove through all my familiar places I saw armored tanks and squads of military police carrying machine guns. Full blocks were gutted, in ashes and smoldering. The smoke from the fires went on for days and days. I considered buying a gun for protection.

But then, I made a decision: I was going to leave L.A. Somehow, I was going to make it happen. And soon.

But where was I going to go? And would Mark even allow me to move, with Sarah?

WHERE TO GO

My mother died on May 30, 1992. Shortly afterward, I began to make my plans to move away from L.A.

My entire family lived in the Bay area, so I considered moving there. But how could I possibly deal with the custody and visitation arrangements? Mark was not about to give up seeing Sarah, especially because he knew it was painful for me to turn her over to him. Even though we were divorced and he was living with Lydia, I could tell he enjoyed causing me emotional pain.

Instead, I chose a place that was far enough away but still within a reasonable — relatively reasonable — driving distance from L.A.

Then, of course, I had to bring up the subject with Mark.

At this point, Sarah was just about 4 years old, so it was a good time to move, before she started kindergarten. The place I chose was a very nice city with a lot to offer in terms of quality of life, and it was also a place that Mark was very familiar with and liked.

I tallied up all the positive reasons why Sarah and I should move to this new city, and I prepared a mental speech for talking with Mark.

How would he react? And what demands would he make?

NO HELP FOR SARAH

Someone asked me recently if, when she was small, Sarah received any counseling for the abuse she suffered.

The short answer is no. And the reason is simple: Mark would not allow it.

Mark and I shared joint legal custody of Sarah, so any decisions about her medical care, for example, had to be agreed to by both of us. If there were an emergency — like if she broke her wrist while at preschool, for example, while in Mark's care (this actually happened) — and she needed urgent medical attention, that was different.

But since Mark denied that Sarah had been abused, either by him or by anyone else, he was not about to let her see a counselor who could possibly corroborate her claims.

That would have been far too risky for him. What if other experts believed her and the evidence began to pile up against him?

And — even more importantly — if she were seeing a counselor, he couldn't keep abusing her.

I had already been reprimanded and threatened with contempt of court if I took Sarah to a counselor without Mark's permission. If I landed in jail, who would protect her then?

TALKING TO MARK

Once I had made the decision that I simply had to move away from LA, I had to talk to Mark about it. Since I had primary physical custody of Sarah, she would live most of the time with me — but he would demand his visitation rights, I was sure of that.

At some level, though, I hoped against hope that maybe, just maybe, he was "through" with us. He had a new girlfriend, whom it seemed like he intended to marry, and I thought perhaps he would start another family and not want to bother with Sarah and me anymore.

How silly that was.

On one of my drop-offs of Sarah at Mark's home, I asked if I could talk to him about something. My heart was racing and I could feel myself starting to feel faint, because I was truly scared about what he might say or do. I only hoped he wouldn't completely blow up. In hindsight, I probably should have had someone there with me. But at the time, it seemed better to not "intimidate" him with anyone else being there — my thought being that he'd be less likely to feel threatened and more likely to acquiesce to my plans if I were there alone.

He heard me out and, as I thought, he approved of the city where I wanted to move. He said he would give some consideration as to how we could alter the visitation schedule so he'd still have the same amount of days during the year, and he'd get back to me.

I knew he was going to talk to his lawyer, and I hoped both of them would have some sense and not try to make things difficult.

I left his house feeling somewhat hopeful, but I was also realistic. I knew I would have to make some sacrifices in order to make this move. I was also nervous about the idea of Sarah being so far away from me when she was with Mark. As it was, in LA our apartment was only a five-minute walk from Mark's house. If we moved, it would be a three-hour drive.

THE ARRANGEMENT

*O*ne of the most surprising things that happened during the summer of 1992 was that Mark actually agreed to "let" me move, with Sarah, to another city.

To do it, though, I had to pay a huge cost.

He agreed to it, yes, but only if we completely rearranged the visitation schedule. After all the divorce and custody proceedings, and after the molestation was ignored by the courts, we were left with sort of a typical arrangement. He saw Sarah every other weekend and one weekend night, and we split the holidays (Christmas every other year, etc.). During the summer, she would stay with him for two weeks, I believe it was — possibly more, I can't quite recall.

Here was the new arrangement:

- Sarah would stay with Mark three weekends out of every four, from Friday night through Sunday afternoon

- Sarah would stay with Mark during every holiday and every birthday; I would not see her for any of them
- Sarah would stay with Mark for six weeks (I believe that's right) during the summer
- I would pay for part of the child care costs for the summer stint

Here was the kicker: Because my lawyers had completely screwed up and did not have anything in our agreement about sharing transportation, Mark forced me to agree to do ALL of the driving.

So three weekends out of four, I was going to have to drive three hours one way, three hours back every Friday night, and three hours one way, three hours back every Sunday night.

I was pretty devastated by these new terms. I felt as though she had been ripped from my arms yet again. I could not protect her from what Mark might do, and she was going to be far away from me.

At the same time, I knew that L.A. was absolutely the wrong place for us to be. I wanted Sarah to live in a place that was prettier, quieter, and far away from Mark — as best as I could make that happen.

I still believed, deep down, that since Mark knew the authorities and I were watching him, he would stop hurting Sarah.

Reluctantly and with great fear, I agreed to the new arrangement. And I made my plans to leave L.A.

Somehow, I thought the literal distance from Mark would help me get better psychologically. I was quite wrong about that. I was wrong about so many things.

THE BODY

The summer of 1992 was the summer my body fell apart.

My mother had died on May 30. I had been dealt a terrible blow by the courts, which refused to protect Sarah from her father's sexual abuse. Financially, I was coping with lawyer bills and no alimony to help pay them, and no permanent job. With all that had been happening in my life, a permanent job had been impossible to even contemplate.

My body started to break down. First, I started hemorrhaging.

I had the menstrual period from hell. It just wouldn't stop, and often it was running like a faucet. I went to two different doctors, who could offer no reason for it and no help for it. I was so desperate I started wearing a diaphragm in addition to tampons and pads to manage it.

After about six or seven weeks, it started to ebb but hadn't completely stopped.

I also was incredibly thin. It wasn't that I didn't want to eat. I literally never even thought about eating. I could go until 2 or 3 o'clock and not even realize that I hadn't eaten that day; I literally never felt hungry. I still have this tendency today: stress makes my appetite disappear completely.

In looking at old photos of myself, I can see that I started to lose weight shortly after Sarah was born. By the time she was 8 or 9 months old, I was much thinner than I had been before her birth.

Several of my friends expressed concern about my weight, and until they said something, I hadn't even noticed. At that point, I didn't address my weight and, frankly, dismissed their concerns.

There were more health problems to come, one of which landed me in the hospital.

Just as the bleeding began to subside (but hadn't quite stopped yet), I developed a new problem. I remember sitting in a movie theater and suddenly feeling a slight pain on my right side, sort of where the lung is. I didn't think much of it at the time because it reminded me of a side stitch you get while running.

But it did not go away. It was constant, and it gradually became worse. Over the next few days, and then a week or more, I began to have trouble doing my normal, daily activities because of the pain.

I went to a couple of doctors. They took x-rays, thinking maybe I had damaged a rib or pulled a muscle. The x-rays showed nothing.

One of the doctors told me, point blank, that the pain was

all in my head. He couldn't figure out what was causing it, therefore it must not be real.

Believe me, it was all too real.

It was nearing the date I was supposed to move to the new city, and I had been dealing with this

pain for about six weeks. It was still getting worse, but I hadn't been able to get any medical help for it.

No painkillers even touched the pain — it was constant, 24 hours a day. Sleep didn't even give me any respite.

One afternoon, I decided to go to the ER in the hospital around the corner. I needed some relief. I drove myself there, but as I stepped out of the car, I collapsed.

I literally could not walk. The entire right side of my torso was on fire with pain, and my right leg felt like it was missing. I screamed as loud as I could for someone to please, please bring a wheelchair.

No one heard me.

On my hands and knees, I crawled to the emergency room entrance.

It was just a few days before I was supposed to move to a new city, one I had chosen because I thought it would be a good place for Sarah to go to school — safer than L.A., prettier than L.A., better than L.A.

But there I was, in the emergency room of a hospital. I couldn't pack up my stuff or do anything to get ready for the move.

I spent about 12 hours in the emergency room before the doctors decided to admit me to the hospital. While I was in the ER, they raised all sorts of possibilities for my problem, including — very scary — a blood clot in my lung. Nope, not it. They were baffled.

All the while, the pain would not subside. A nurse administered morphine, then came back 30 minutes later, looked at me and said, "It's not working at all, is it?" She gave me more. Came back. Asked me again.

I shook my head "no," because by this point I literally couldn't speak without screaming. I had given the hospital staff my dad's phone number so he could drive to L.A. (a 7-hour trip) and help me.

The hospital staff finally found a medicine that worked for the pain — a highly addictive narcotic that I'm sure they would've rather avoided giving me. Eventually, they admitted me to the hospital to run more tests to see what the hell was causing this pain.

My dad found me by following my screams down the hallway. When they admitted me, they did not yet have a doctor's authorization to continue administering the pain medication. When the ER dose wore off, the agony was indescribable.

For six days, I struggled to deal with the innumerable tests they put me through. Some required me not to eat for 24 hours, which was doubly bad because I was already thin and the pain medication was wreaking havoc on my digestive system.

At the end of the sixth day, the doctor — Dr. Incompetence, I called him — sent a psychiatrist in to see me.

Before he even said anything, I told him, "I'm sure you're a very good psychiatrist and want to help me. But I assure you, this pain is not psychosomatic. It is being caused by something, and no amount of talking is going to make it go away." And I sent him packing.

On the seventh day, Dr. Incompetence ordered an MRI.

Within minutes of my return to my hospital room after completing the MRI, he rushed in. I have never in my life heard such a sincere apology from a doctor.

Turns out I had a herniated disc in my spine that was pressing on the nerve bundle. It may have also been the cause of the hemorrhaging I had had a few weeks earlier, he said.

By this time, my family — my sister, her husband, and my dad — had packed my stuff for me and moved it to my new city. I had no more time to spend with Dr. Incompetence.

On day 8, I checked myself out, against the wishes of Dr. Incompetence. I also stopped the narcotic cold turkey, which is probably one of the dumbest things I've ever done.

My dad picked me up and drove me to my new city, to the new apartment he and I had found a few weeks before. I could walk, but barely. I immediately started going into withdrawals from the medication — I literally looked like a heroin addict going through detox — and I dropped even more weight. The veins in my arms throbbed as if they were on fire (which would continue for 6 weeks).

I felt broken. But for reasons I cannot explain, I also felt a surge of hope.

TRAUMA'S HEALTH EFFECTS

I have no doubt that the trauma I experienced living with Mark, and the subsequent trauma and stress of dealing with his sexual abuse of our daughter, had — and continue to have — a major negative effect on my health.

Interestingly, this doesn't seem to be a topic that's discussed very often related to domestic violence.

For me, the problems with my back, which continued for the next several years, and my overall poor immune system seem obviously related to the stress I endured for such a long time.

I've since learned that other physical conditions and some forms of cancer seem more pronounced in women who have endured domestic violence.

It's not "just" the psychological and emotional effects that can become debilitating, it's also the physical effects.

Sometimes it surprises me that I've managed to live as well as I have, all things considered. A day doesn't go by, though, where I don't notice a remnant of the abuse: a distinctly negative reaction to hearing yelling (not uncommon where I currently live, in a big city); a fear of losing something important, like documents (because Mark played some intense head games with me about that); and so many other things.

There are days when I feel like an empty shell whose life simply squeezed out of her and walked away, disappearing into the sand.

"YOU BLAME ME"

On one of my visits to pick up Sarah from Mark's house, he said something that stunned me. It came from out of nowhere, and I have no idea why he said it.

With some help from Lydia, Sarah was getting her things together to come back home with me. It was a Sunday evening, and by that point I had already driven the 6-hour round trip to their home on Friday, another 3 hours to come pick her up on Sunday, and I had the final 3 hours ahead of me to get back home.

The driving was brutal.

Usually Sarah and I stopped at some point for food, like In-n-Out burgers. Other times, if she was asleep in the car I would just force myself to keep driving so we could get home faster.

As difficult as the driving was, I found a positive aspect to it: it really allowed us to have several uninterrupted hours together, so we could talk about anything and everything. I often feel like those drives brought us closer together.

So it was a Sunday, and I was just ready to be home. I was standing in the dining area with Mark, and I could hear Sarah and Lydia in Sarah's bedroom, putting her things back in her bag and chatting away.

Suddenly, Mark turned to me and said, "You blame me, don't you? You blame me for the miscarriage. You think I caused it."

I stared blankly at him for a moment, not sure if I should answer for fear of provoking an angry response. But then I said it.

"Yes, I do."

He nodded his head. And that was that.

Sarah and Lydia emerged, and Sarah and I left, got in the car, and took the same route we drove the day I left Mark. It all felt very familiar, but not in a good way.

HER SCREAMS

To this very day, to this very moment, I can still hear her screams as if they're happening right now.

On one of the drives back to our new town, after I picked her up at Mark's, Sarah was very quiet, and then she fell asleep.

This was unusual behavior for her. Usually she was hungry — sometimes Mark didn't give her dinner before I picked her up — so we'd stop for food. And often she liked to tell me about her pets that she had at Mark's house.

But on this drive, she didn't say much of anything and nodded off before I even realized it. She started to wake up when we arrived at our home, but she still wasn't talking.

I brought her inside, and suddenly, it started. The screams.

All she did was scream. And scream. And scream.

By this time, she was 4-1/2 years old and was very verbal — she already knew how to read — so when she wouldn't talk, I knew something had to be wrong.

I thought at first she was in physical pain, but she wouldn't answer my questions. I decided I needed to look her over, so I began looking for cuts or bruises. I saw nothing out of the ordinary.

She kept screaming.

After about 20 minutes, I called my dad and told him what was going on. I couldn't get Sarah to calm down. I took her to her room, gave her all the things that usually comforted her — blankets and stuff toys, and our own cat, Candy — but nothing was working. My dad was very concerned, as was I.

He asked me if I had looked for any obvious signs of sexual abuse. I told him I had not, but I thought maybe if I put her into a warm bath, she might calm down. While bathing her, I could perhaps look for any overt signs that she'd been hurt by Mark.

So I put her into a warm bath and did my best to look without causing any fear or anxiety.

She continued screaming. Literally, it was nonstop. Screaming, crying, until she was almost blue in the face.

I saw nothing physically wrong with her.

The bath did nothing to help her calm down. So after about 5 minutes, I took her out, wrapped her in a towel, and brought her into her bedroom. I helped her get into some PJ's, all while she was still screaming.

After a full hour, she was so worn down by the physical requirements of screaming, she started to fall asleep.

And when she fell asleep, the screaming finally stopped. But her sobs went on for hours, literally hours.

I never was able to determine what happened. The next day I tried to bring it up, but she did not want to talk about anything. Remembering the judge's admonishment — that if I took her to a counselor again without Mark's permission, I could be held in contempt of court and Sarah could be taken from me — I struggled with what to do.

So I did my best, as her mother, to watch her behavior and let her know that she could talk to me about anything, anything at all.

It was many more years before she finally broke her silence.

FATIGUE

~~~

I have never known such fatigue. The driving, all the driving ... it was absolutely exhausting. Several times on my way home from taking Sarah to LA, I thought for sure I was going to fall asleep. More than once, I pulled off the freeway to sleep for 30 minutes, usually in a specific church parking lot that became my own personal rest stop — it seemed like a safe place.

I listened to music, to talk radio, to whatever. I didn't have a cell phone until a couple of years into the driving, so I couldn't talk to anyone when I was alone in the car. Hours upon hours in the car, driving on California freeways, took a toll on me, infusing my body with a permanent state of weariness.

While the time alone with Sarah was nice and we were able to talk, the drive on the way home from dropping her off at Mark's house was not only interminable, it was emotionally draining. I hated — hated — leaving her with Mark. I prayed and prayed that Mark wasn't abusing Sarah, and I kept a close eye on her and looked for any sign, no matter how small, that would indicate that the abuse had continued.

Oftentimes I would find myself crying on that solo drive back home. Before I realized it, I would be sobbing and, once again, would have to pull off the road to collect myself so I could continue.

The worry and the anxiety over Sarah's safety, combined with the fatigue, made these drives almost like a form of torture.

RAPE / FORGIVENESS

*D*uring our marriage, every time Mark and I had sex, it was rape.

After our honeymoon and the rape he committed against me, I never wanted to sleep with him again. But because he was someone who was supposed to love and care for me, my emotions became extremely conflicted and confused. I didn't know what to do, I didn't know who to talk to about it, and I was afraid of him.

Sometimes the rape was preceded by a violent act or a threat of it. Sometimes it wasn't. But the thing is, once someone instills that kind of fear — literally, the fear that you might die if you don't comply — violence, per se, isn't necessary for you to believe you must do as he says. All Mark had to do was look at me a certain way, and I knew trouble would be coming if I didn't do what he wanted. After Sarah was born, of course my fear was magnified: now if I didn't comply, he could hurt our child if he wanted to (which of course he did, even though I didn't know about it).

I never thought seriously about going to the police. I mean, what would I have said to them? I didn't think anyone would believe me. In fact, I'm sure they wouldn't have. Without obvious evidence, whom do you think they would believe?

The psychological damage of seven years of rape is still present in my life today. It's difficult to describe the depth of the violation one feels. For me, it's as if someone put a shotgun to my belly and pulled the trigger, but I'm still walking and talking, working and living. There is a gigantic hole that can never been fully healed. So I've learned to live with the emptiness there and have tried to fill it with other things, like love for my daughter and for the people in my life who do truly care about me.

For many victims of crime, forgiveness is part of their healing. I'm not so magnanimous. Despite my spiritual beliefs in the value of forgiveness, I have not forgiven Mark for what he did to me and to Sarah. Perhaps if I could forgive him, that emptiness inside would disappear. But it might not.

In order to forgive Mark for raping me, hurting me, abusing me, and molesting Sarah, I would have to find some sort of excuse for him, and for his behavior: like, He had a bad childhood, or, He is mentally ill, or He doesn't know right from wrong, or … whatever.

There is no excuse. He did all of it because he could, because he wanted to, because it suited him. There may be many underlying reasons for his behavior, but I don't care about any of that. He knew exactly what he was doing.

How can one forgive someone like that? And how, exactly, would that make me feel any better, anyway? Yes, I still carry some anger.

Forgiveness is not the only replacement emotion for anger. And I'm not so sure that completely letting go of that anger is a good thing, either.

HALFWAY / HEADACHES

After awhile — I'm not exactly sure how long, perhaps one or two years into it — Mark agreed to meet me at the halfway point. Not on every drive, mind you, but at least once, maybe twice a month.

This was a relief to me, but at the same time it meant that I could not see the state of the house as often as I would have liked. But that was a small price to pay for some help with the driving.

Mark sometimes met me on his own, sometimes he brought Lydia. Every time was awkward. If it was just Mark, we would occasionally try to make small talk. I'd ask about his family, about his work. He'd sometimes ask about my life, but not very often. If Lydia were with him, again I'd try to talk with her.

She was friendly enough, but we never connected in any real way.

We'd meet in a nice little park, across from a zoo that

Mark would sometimes take Sarah to. All this time, she managed to keep a good attitude about riding in the car.

After a few months of doing these drives, however, Sarah started to develop headaches. Nearly every time we did a drive, she'd get a headache. It wasn't carsickness, it was truly a headache.

Then, nearly every time we rode in the car even at home, she'd get a headache. If it was more than five or ten minutes in the car, BAM — headache.

I began to wonder why this was happening, whether it was some sort of psychosomatic response.

Now, I believe it was. I think it was a reaction to stress, because I believe she was feeling the same level of stress I did when I had to be around Mark. The body can only cope with so much before it starts to rebel. And in Sarah's case, it was with headaches.

SO MANY BIRTHDAYS

I missed so many birthdays, and Thanksgivings, and Christmases. Sarah spent them all with Mark, just so she and I could have a separate life in a new city, away from L.A.

But I knew that even if I stayed in L.A., Sarah would still be with Mark, unprotected and alone. There was nothing I could do about that — the court had seen to it that my child would be locked in a relationship with her abusive father.

On one of Sarah's birthdays, I think when she turned six, Mark "allowed" me to come down to L.A. to see her for a while. I picked her up at his house and took her to a nearby park, and I gave her a present: a kite that we could fly together. We played and flew the kite for about an hour or so, and then I had to take her back to Mark's for her party.

The depth of pain I felt was indescribable when I said good bye to her, every single time — not just on her birthday that year. The longing was physically debilitating, as if someone took a baseball bat to my knees.

I know there were things she liked about being with Mark. Because no matter what their parents do to them, children still love them, deep down. And if all they saw were the bad things in their relationship, it would be difficult to go on living.

Mark was generous with gifts, he enjoyed cooking and made Sarah all her favorite foods, and he went all out when it came to decorating the house at Christmastime, for example. He had a swimming pool, and he bought her a dog — things she did not have with me.

But all those years, all those birthdays … and things were happening in that household that I didn't know about, couldn't know about. Although she gave me a huge hint one day. And I missed it.

PART V

NEVER-ENDING NIGHTMARE

At one point in my life, at age 33, after my divorce but during the trauma that followed it, I considered suicide.

The weird thing is, though, I didn't feel depressed. I thought about Julian and remembered how he behaved when he was depressed – trying to jump out of the car, hiding in his room and not answering calls, not changing his clothes or showering for several days – and I knew I wasn't truly depressed.

I went to see a counselor, and she agreed that I was not depressed; in fact, I hadn't had the kinds of thoughts a truly suicidal person would have. I hadn't thought about how I would do it, or when, or if I'd leave a note. It was more like I was exploring my options, if you will.

I remember one visit to the counselor, in particular. (I was only allowed 6 visits under my insurance plan, so I had to make them count.) The counselor walked me through a guided imagery session to try and help me find the intestinal fortitude I needed to deal with my current life situation.

In that guided imagery, I remember imagining that inside my belly was a safe place for me to hide when things got rough. I could go there and curl up, just as I did before I was born, and relax into a soothing water bath. I could have other comforts there, too. I remember saying that I wanted to have a blanket with me, so I would never be cold. And I wanted to be able to hear birds singing, too. All those things were possible inside this incredibly safe place.

I needed a safe place, even if it was just in my own mind. At that time, I was having to see Mark, now my ex-husband, several times a month as we exchanged our daughter for visitations. But it was not just the seeing him that unnerved me and knowing that my daughter was going to stay with such a monstrous person.

It was that I knew what else was going on in that house, and I was literally powerless to stop it, save from taking my daughter and leaving the country. (Believe me, I contemplated that option several times.)

Of all the terrible things that happened to me during my marriage, nothing prepared me, or even warned me, about the possibility that Mark would ever truly harm our daughter.

Sometimes, I felt as if I wasn't worthy of living. After all, I had brought her into this world, into this household, chosen this man as her father. And what was happening to her while she was there seemed like it was all my fault.

Do I realize now that it wasn't? No, not completely. Despite what lawyers and police and counselors have said to me over the years — that there was nothing I could have done — I still believe, deep down, that I could have prevented it from happening.

That thought will be with me until the day I die. Thankfully, though, I want that day to be a long time from now.

MOLESTATION = MANY FORMS

One thing I came to realize during all of this horror was that child molestation comes in many forms, and a lot of those are not discussed in those "good touch, bad touch" sessions they teach kids in school.

Because the fact is, sexual molestation does not have to involve touch at all. It can mean exposing children to pornography.

It can mean having sex in front of children, or in bed with them.

It can mean creating a highly sexualized environment, where sex is demonstrated openly in a way that the child cannot comprehend: all in an effort to scare them into eventual compliance with the adults' sexual demands.

It can mean talking to a child in a sexual and provocative way.

It can mean a PARENT does all of these things. Not a stranger. A PARENT.

When you're not a child molester, you don't think like a child molester. So I didn't think of any of these scenarios (and I'm sure there are plenty more).

It never dawned on me that any of this behavior was going on, because my idea of sexual molestation/incest was much too narrow. I was still looking for signs that matched what Sarah had revealed to me when she was younger.

Instead, when she was about 10 years old, Sarah told me about something that, on the face of it, seemed ... not all that unusual.

I was wrong. I just didn't know it, at the time.

At that time, my new husband, Jim, and I had been married for about a year.

Sarah was adjusting quite well to having a stepdad, and Jim was doing a good job of blending into what had been a mother-daughter family unit, which was pretty strong after nearly 7 years of being on our own.

By this time, Mark and Lydia had gotten married — they dated for four years first — and Sarah was still going to their home regularly, as always. The ridiculous schedule had remained the same, only now I had some help with the driving and Mark and Lydia met us halfway most of the time.

One night when I was putting Sarah to bed, she told me, very nervously, that she was frightened at Mark's house because he and Lydia made love very loudly at night, and it made it difficult for her to sleep.

When Sarah told me this, I wasn't particularly alarmed. I knew the two bedrooms at the house were close together, separated only by a bathroom, so it seemed reasonable that this could be a problem. I did wonder, though, how long this had been going on — although I didn't press Sarah on that point.

I listened to what Sarah had to say, and I tried to read between the lines. I did not see anything that raised a red flag, only that she was having the problem she described.

Of course, Jim knew all about what had happened with Mark — I had told him everything.

To be on the safe side, though, I made an executive decision, as they call it: I was going to take Sarah to a counselor

And I wasn't going to tell Mark! Courts be damned this time. It was 7 years later — 7 years after the ruling that gave her over to Mark on a regular basis, without anyone there to be sure she was safe, despite all the evidence to the contrary.

So I took Sarah to see a counselor that I had been to myself a few times, a very nice woman named Michelle. I had told Michelle beforehand what had happened to Sarah, and I asked her to please look for any signs of abuse that I might not be able to see.

We went to see Michelle a few times, and Michelle told me (privately) that she didn't see anything obvious regarding current sexual abuse. When it came to dealing with the problem at hand, the only thing we could think to do was to give Sarah a Walkman-type device, so she could block out the noise and listen to her favorite music at night.

I bought her a bunch of CD's, and together with what she already had, she had quite a collection to take in her travel CD case when she went to Mark's house.

This solution seemed to work for a little while.

Until it didn't. Only I didn't know it wasn't working until nearly a year later.

When Sarah and I went to see the counselor, Michelle, we discussed the possibility of my talking to Mark and Lydia about this problem.

Knowing our history, however, Michelle advised against it. Since we had no evidence of anything else going on, she thought — considering Mark's personality — that it would be seen as aggressive, possibly putting Sarah in more danger.

I agreed.

The last thing I wanted to do was provoke a confrontation with Mark, to put him on the defensive in any way.

I know how this sounds, as if we were kowtowing to Mark and allowing him to be in control. There are times, however, when you have to make a decision that is in your own personal best interests, in terms of safety. I wasn't willing to risk our safety, or Sarah's safety, by confronting him: because that is how he would have viewed any conversation about this situation.

And frankly, I couldn't imagine actually having a conversation like that with Mark: Excuse me, but you and Lydia make love too loudly and it disturbs Sarah. Could you tone it down?

Under the circumstances, that was out of the question.

I didn't realize it at the time, but that conversation was going to happen. Just not in the way I expected.

JIM

I met Jim at work, at a time in my life when I had really determined that I did not want to get married to anyone. In the few years after leaving Mark, I had had three relationships, but they were all disastrous.

Mostly, I was choosing men with serious problems, like cheating or alcoholism.

Jim embodied everything you'd expect from a "good man." He was nice and polite, and he showed me respect. His dark hair and warm eyes, combined with a genuine kindness and firm, hugging grip — he had been a star athlete and was still in excellent shape -- made me feel safe, and rightly so. We felt a strong connection almost right away, and although I wasn't in a hurry to move the relationship along quickly, it did so on its own.

After six months of dating, Jim moved into our condo. Six months later, we were married. I trusted Jim, and he has never given me any reason not to. He has never harmed me in any way.

We have been married for 14 years now, but the marriage has been fraught with problems. I told him recently that if I had known the extent of the damage done to my mind and spirit by Mark, I never would have gotten married again, to anyone.

There are times when I wonder if I shouldn't end it, for Jim's sake. At 51, he's still young enough — and definitely still attractive enough — to have a good life with someone else.

I don't know if our marriage will survive. We do love each other, but often I think it's simply not enough. With time, and with continued therapeutic help, I might be able to become the marriage partner I want to be.

SAM

Sarah became very attached to her cat at Mark's house, named Sam. Sam was a black cat, very fluffy, and he was super friendly and sweet. Even more, he loved to be cuddled and held. Imagine a living stuffed animal you could hold next to you at night, and that was Sam.

During the nights when Sarah felt afraid at Mark's house, she pushed her Walkman headphones into her ears and clutched Sam close to her. And she cried.

I had no idea any of this was going on, of course. She had told me she was terribly frightened at night at Mark's house, because Mark and Lydia made a lot of noise when they were making love. We tried to deal with that in the best way we could think of, with the Walkman.

She didn't tell me any of this about Sam and the crying until much later, when we realized that her fears were about much more than loud lovemaking.

Sarah learned about Sam's death in a letter from Mark. He

told her that one day, he went into her room and Sam was on the floor, not moving. Sam had simply died in his sleep.

Sarah was devastated. She cried and cried and cried. And she kept asking me, "How could something so beautiful, like Sam, ever die, Mom? How could that happen?"

Like many questions that arose in those days, I had no answer that would satisfy her, or me.

CLOSER TO THE TRUTH

In spring of 2000 — 9-1/2 years after I moved out, and 6-1/2 years after I moved to a new city with Sarah — we were nearing school vacation time. Sarah was 11 years old and in 6th grade.

Even though I was remarried, Mark refused to alter the visitation arrangements so we could have her with us for some of the holidays. Sarah was still with Mark and his family on Thanksgiving, Christmas, her birthday, all school breaks, and several weeks during the summer. We had to celebrate our holidays together on dates of our own design.

Spring break was coming up, and as usual, Mark and Lydia had planned to take Sarah on a trip with them. I believe they were going to Palm Springs that year — they had gone there on spring break the previous year.

About a month before spring break, Sarah was supposed to go to Mark and Lydia's for her usual weekend visit. It was … maybe a Wednesday before she would go there on Friday.

That night, I was in Sarah's room as she was getting into bed and was about to say "good night" to her. She got under the covers and suddenly got very quiet.

"Mom," she said, "I don't want to go to my dad's house this weekend." She started to cry.

I held her in my arms as she told me about not only how loud their lovemaking was, but it was to the point of raucous. She explained how she held Sam, her cat, and cried and she tried to drown out the noise with the music in her headphones.

She also described Mark and Lydia's behavior outside the bedroom as overly sexualized. "He's always grabbing her boobs and her butt and saying sexual stuff," she told me.

I could see she was upset and, frankly, traumatized by what she had seen and heard. I let her finish telling me about it — and at that moment, it's as far as the conversation went, that she was upset about listening to them at night and seeing their behavior with each other during the day.

I helped her get to sleep and then came downstairs to talk to my husband, Jim.

We made a decision: The two of us were going to drive to the usual meeting place on Friday night, without Sarah, and talk to Mark and Lydia about what she had said. We believed — or at least, we hoped — we could have a civil conversation about the situation.

So that Friday night, we drove to the meeting place and rehearsed, over and over again in the car, what we were going to say to them. We did not expect the reaction we got. Never in a million years.

MEETING

When my husband Jim and I met Mark and Lydia without Sarah in the car, of course they knew immediately that something was up.

I remember feeling so nervous about talking to them that my teeth were chattering.

It was a beautiful spring day, in this city in California on the beach. We always met in a park, and since it was sunny, I tried to find us a spot in the shade in which to talk.

I wish I could remember the exact words that were spoken. What I do remember is standing across from Mark and Lydia and telling them — Jim and I sort of alternating between us — what Sarah had said.

The upshot, of course, was that she didn't want to go to their house that weekend, which is why she was at home and we were there in the park, talking to them.

I stared into Mark's face to see if I could find any hint of anger. He was doing a good job of controlling it, but it was definitely there. He interrupted us occasionally, as though he couldn't quite contain himself.

But he did not show his anger overtly. It was under the surface.

As for Lydia, she was openly upset about what we were telling her. At least, that's how it seemed at the time. She started to cry and said that she was sorry Sarah was feeling uncomfortable at their house, that she would never want her to feel that way, and so forth.

We told them that we had tried to solve the problem by giving her a Walkman and headphones, which they told us they were aware of. But clearly, that wasn't solving the problem.

I'm not sure how long we talked. My mind was floating elsewhere while my body shook in the California sunlight and tried to stay present.

The conversation ended with them saying they would go home and think things through, and we would see if Sarah would like to talk to them over the phone. We also mentioned that we wanted to take Sarah to see a counselor (Michelle, who had helped us secretly before), and they seemed fine with that.

On the drive home, Jim and I remarked that the whole thing actually went better than we ever anticipated. No one got angry, there were no accusations made by either side, and they seemed to understand what we were telling them. When we got home, we told Sarah what happened, and while she was still anxious about everything, she seemed happy to know that she did not have to go there and could decide when she was ready to talk to them on the phone.

So everything seemed relatively OK to us, all things considered. Holy s*&t, were we ever wrong. W R O N G.

LOSS

Recovering from being in a violent relationship is not easy. Recovery is compounded when there are children involved, because clearly your focus has to be on them, not on yourself.

It's only now, with my daughter grown up, that I have been able to start really working on my recovery. It is work.

Today, I'm struggling with allowing myself to feel the intense grief over so much terrible loss. It's different from losing a person who has died. I've lost my mother, my father, my mother-in-law, friends and other people close to me. With each one of those deaths, the grief has been painful, but the loss was palpable. Simply put, I didn't — couldn't — see them anymore. They were buried or cremated, there was a ceremony around that, and they were clearly gone.

It has not been simple to grieve for them, but the loss itself was fairly easy to define. With what I've experienced with Mark, it's not so easy to define. What did I lose?

- My youth
- My husband, the man I thought I married, and the life I thought we would have
- My sense of security
- My belief that when someone marries you, they truly want to be your partner — it was absolutely shattered on my wedding night
- My trust in other people, which I've tried to regain
- My belief in myself and even basic knowledge of who I am
- My dreams and any goals I might have had as a young person; I have no connection to them whatsoever and don't remember what they were
- My daughter's father
- My daughter's father's family
- My innocence
- My daughter's innocence

I'm sure as I sit with this grief, I will realize even more aspects of myself and my life that I've lost. It's the actual "sitting" with the grief that is so difficult. It feels like I'm drowning under Niagara Falls, every hour of every day. The moment I think the grief is gone, I'll see something — a young woman smiling broadly, enjoying a moment with friends in a restaurant, or a mother with a young baby girl — and it all floods back again.

EX PARTE

An ex parte motion is what it's called when one party files a motion with the court without much notice to the other party.

In other words, it's a slimeball tactic to get a judge to make a quick ruling without benefit of the other side having any representation.

We had met with Mark and Lydia in the park on Friday.

On Monday afternoon around 4 pm, I got a voicemail message on my answering machine. It was Mark's attorney. Mark had filed an ex parte motion with the court, and the court was going to hear it on Wed. Mind you, he filed it in Los Angeles County court, and I lived 200 miles away from there. I had no lawyer where I lived, and I certainly didn't have a lawyer anymore in Los Angeles. (I wouldn't have considered using my previous attorneys, who were, frankly, incompetent.)

I couldn't even comprehend what was happening.

Mark was filing suit against me for violating our visitation agreement. Yes, that's right. For violating our visitation agreement.

We met Mark and Lydia in the park that prior Friday and explained that Sarah was not comfortable going there, considering their raucous lovemaking and other overly sexual behavior. And this is what Mark decided to do. Go on the offense.

Jim and I went into panic mode. We simply had to have someone in court to represent us. And we needed to find someone FAST.

I can't remember exactly how it came about, but we made a flurry of calls to people we knew who either were lawyers or who knew lawyers. We found a lawyer in our city — again, can't remember exactly how — who said she knew a family lawyer in Los Angeles, and she'd call him for us right away. His name was Peter.

We waited by the phone for Peter to call us, which he did. I told him the situation, and I gave him all the information that was left on the answering machine.

He said he would represent us.

Tuesday was an insane day, trying to get money to Peter's law firm to get things started, filling him in on all the details he might need in court the following day, and on and on.

But what happened Tuesday night changed everything.

BEDTIME

Sarah obviously knew something was going on, because Jim and I were running around like maniacs trying to get legal representation. We had a little more than a day to find someone, which was tough considering we were about 200 miles from the L.A. County courthouse, in a completely different city!

We managed to find an attorney who worked in L.A. at a reputable small firm, who came recommended by a good attorney in our town. But really, how many choices did we have? We needed someone, anyone, so we could hear exactly what Mark was suing us for — I could not believe it was simply because Sarah wouldn't visit him one weekend. One weekend, out of eight years.

Tuesday night at bedtime, the night before the ex parte hearing, I sat down with Sarah and talked to her about exactly what was happening. She was 11-1/2 years old, old enough to understand.

I told her again that when Jim and I met with them on the weekend and discussed our concerns, everything seemed to go fairly well. I really was confused about why Mark would go on the offense like this — it didn't make sense to me.

Sarah started to cry. And cry, and cry.

She told me everything. Everything that had been going on all those years: the "games" that Mark played with her so he could touch her private parts, the traumatic exposure to his and Lydia's sexual escapades, including having intercourse openly in a hotel room in the bed right next to her.

She went into detail about their overtly sexual behavior at home, basically engaging in sexual conduct over and over again in front of her.

On the spring break vacation the previous year, things got even more serious. Not only did Mark and Lydia have sex in front of Sarah, when they were finished, Mark put his underwear back on and lay in bed next to Sarah (Lydia had left the room to go to the bathroom).

He looked at Sarah, then looked down at his private parts, then back at her as if to say, "Do you want some?" or "Pretty soon, you'll get it, too."

She lived in fear all the time she was with him — just like I did.

As she was talking, I realized that all these years, all these years, he had continued the sexual abuse in one way or another, grooming her to become one of his sexual partners. She mentioned a lot of other things that led me to believe — 100 percent — that he would eventually rape her.

I had to get this information to Peter before the court appearance the next day. Everything depended on it.

LETTER TO MARK

Mark,

There are times when I wish you had killed me

... during one of your rages, in the years before Sarah was born. Maybe you could have hit my head with something you threw across the room. Or one of the times you grabbed me and pushed me, I could have fallen and broken my neck. Or you could have decided to drown me in the pool, made it look like an accident.

But the truth is, you did kill me.

I'm still walking around, but I've been dead ever since the first night of our marriage, when you raped me.

I was exhausted from the late-night wedding, and I needed to rest. But you wouldn't take no for an answer. You held me down, and in your eyes I saw no love at all. Just rage, and hate, and the power enough to kill me.

The me I knew before that night is dead. She resides only in so *many old photo albums, and in the way I imagine her sometimes when I allow myself to daydream about her. She was a beautiful person, inside and out: someone who could have had a wonderful life, full of love and accomplishments.*

I wish you could know what it's like to live, but not. I wouldn't wish that on anyone else. Only you. Because you have a special place in my life.

You are my murderer. And I am your victim.

And when you harmed our daughter the way you did, you started to kill her, too. But I stopped you. Thanks to me, and to her own inner strength, not only is she still alive, but she is living.

No matter how many more hours, or days, or years you and I see the light of day, you will always be my murderer, and I will always be your victim. You carved that honorary place for yourself into my flesh.

Lucy

SARAH'S DISCLOSURE, AND MINE

When Sarah told me what had happened to her, about the abuse and terror she was suffering at the hands of her father and his wife, she and I were in her bedroom, getting her into bed.

It was a cute room on the second floor of our house, with a slanted ceiling and a view out the back toward some other homes and the surrounding hills. I had painted the walls a happy yellow, at her request, and I put some neon stars on the ceiling that glowed in the dark.

We lived in a rural area, where the only noises at night were crickets and frogs, and in the early morning we could hear the trains chugging by. It was an idyllic, peaceful home.

That peace was shattered by her words and punctuated by her sobbing. She couldn't seem to stop crying. I knew that she must have been terribly afraid to tell me everything; Mark must have made it clear that she should never talk to me about any of this.

I also told her something important.

After she finished, I told her what had happened when she was a toddler. I explained everything: about what had happened to her — the abuse and how she told me about it — and about the court system, the ruling, all of it.

I assured her that things would be different this time. Even though I knew it was going to get ugly, I also knew that the outcome would be different. I would make it so.

Sarah listened to me, knowingly. For the truth was, I was telling her something she, of course, already knew. Because it had happened to her.

When I finally got her calmed down that night, I tucked her into bed with the blankets my mother had knitted for her, and a little quilt I had made with fabric depicting the stars, the moon and the planets — she's always loved looking at the stars.

ALL OVER AGAIN

It felt as if we were jettisoned back to 1991-'92.

Suddenly, we were back in the court system, fighting for Sarah's safety and feeling the full weight of the "authorities" against us. Walking uphill pushing a boulder would have been easier to do. The sensation was one of pure oppression.

I continually asked myself — and I do it still, today — "Why is it so difficult to protect a child from abuse?"

Nothing had changed since the first time we went through all of this, except that Sarah was much older (11 instead of nearly 3) and could understand the implications of everything that was happening. She knew that it was deadly serious, and that what had happened to her could pose serious consequences to Mark and Lydia.

As before, we talked to the police, social workers, psychologists, lawyers. We made court appearances. We took depositions.

We begged relatives to loan us money and nearly had to file bankruptcy anyway.

Emotionally, I swirled among so many feelings: déjà vu, fear, anxiety, sadness, bereavement, and of course, anger. There were times I wished Mark would just die, so it would all be over with.

Any healing that I had done for myself by this point, which in all honesty was not all that much, was crushed by this wave of nauseating truth: that my daughter, despite all my best efforts to protect her, had been hurt AGAIN by her father — and her stepmother, to add to the horror. (She used to be a nanny, for God's sake! I pitied the poor children who had been in her care.)

This time — this time — the outcome simply had to be different. No matter what it took, I was never, ever going to allow Mark near Sarah again.

POLICE

*P*art of the process of dealing with child molestation is talking to the police. This time, we spoke to the police about two separate things: first, we wanted to know if what had happened to Sarah in Palm Springs the year before constituted a crime that could be prosecuted.

Second, the police interviewed Sarah at length, out of my presence, and also spoke to my current husband, Jim and me.

On the first count, the police said that — does this sound familiar? — while a crime may have been committed, there was no physical evidence to back it up. It was her word against his.

When I heard that wording coming from the police officers, I had all I could do not to vomit on the spot. I remember that my husband, my father and my brother were there with me for support while I dealt with the police. They were furious, and while we had to keep our heads on straight

— we were at a police station, after all — the heat of our anger was palpable.

To their credit, the officers said they understood our feelings. Maybe they did, intellectually.

I, on the other hand, began to feel as though I was trapped in some nightmarish episode of "The Twilight Zone," where I am damned to live the same wretched life over and over again.

The police were of no use to us, except that they determined Sarah was not lying about what had happened to her. Neither were Jim or I. We were all telling the truth.

Well, they said the same thing when she was 3 years old, too. Was that supposed to make me feel better? Was it supposed to reassure me in some way?

DR. CHEN

Another step — here we go again — was talking to a psychologist. This time, it was a woman, Dr. Chen, who conducted the initial psychiatric evaluations.

Backing up for a moment, the court deemed, as it is wont to do, that all of us should be examined by a psychologist: we would do a personality inventory (the MMPI), for example, and other psychological testing — ink blots and such, plus a session with the psychologist.

During this time, Mark and Lydia were not allowed to see Sarah, as put forth in a temporary order by the judge. However, a social worker had deemed Jim and I to be fit enough parents so that she was not removed from our home during the process. (Can you even imagine what that would have done to her?)

The judge ordered that this first evaluation be conducted by Dr. Chen, whose office was actually located near the city in which we lived, not in L.A. So Mark and Lydia had to make a

3-hour drive to their appointment — which didn't bother me one bit, after all those years of my driving to LA and back!

Dr. Chen was a very perceptive, straight-shooting type of psychologist. She didn't mince words. We did all the exams, and she came back to us with this: that what Sarah, Jim and I were saying about Mark and Lydia's behavior was, in her estimation, absolutely true.

However, she told us that in her opinion, Mark and Lydia could be helped by going to a counselor. She also said that Mark could possibly be aided by certain medications and — if he were motivated — could change his behavior.

I wanted so much to believe her. Let me repeat that.

I wanted so much to believe her.

For in all the years since I had left Mark, I had never stopped hoping that maybe, just maybe, he would value his daughter enough to get help for himself, so that their relationship could somehow be "normal."

But Mark's idea of "normal" could never be translated into a life where Sarah, or I, or any reasonable person could exist.

SHOCKING INFORMATION ABOUT MARK

What Dr. Chen and the rest of us didn't know at the time was that Mark's family — mother, father, and his three sisters (all older than he) — was severely, severely dysfunctional.

Yes, as I have written before, I thought there was domestic violence going on between his parents. And yes, at one point I even suspected that his two young nieces (two of Sarah's cousins) were being molested by someone, although that was long before I had reason to suspect Mark, and later, I never had any proof that he was involved.

What I found out in 2009 was that incest likely was part of his childhood experiences.

One of those nieces of Mark's that I just mentioned is still close with Sarah; they are cousins, but they are almost like sisters. Of all of Mark's relatives, she's the only one with whom Sarah has any regular contact. She's a lovely young woman who has had her share of difficulties, too.

In 2009, she told Sarah (who then told me) that at the family Thanksgiving dinner, Mark's middle sister Lynn – the one who originally introduced me to Mark – got very, very upset and started to recount, loudly and assuredly, all the things that made their family so terrible.

Sarah's cousin said she sat there at the dinner table, in disbelief, as Mark's sister described her sexual encounters with Mark, which he apparently did not deny.

The sister who had introduced me to Mark, the one whose apartment we often visited before we were married, had apparently been a sexual partner of Mark's during their teen years. And we're not just talking about heavy petting; it went as far as intercourse, more than once, according to Lynn's Thanksgiving dinner rant.

It sounds crazy. In any other case, I might not believe it to be true. But deep down, I know that it is. Everything makes sense now.

I always sensed a strong connection between Mark and this particular sister. It was a little weird and, frankly, it made me uncomfortable years ago, long before I knew all of this. He spent a lot of time with Lynn, stayed over at her apartment often before he and I were married (and even after, rarely). While there was never anything overtly sexual about their relationship, it just all seemed … odd.

Mark was always incredibly generous with her. Gave her money, even bought drugs for her once (she had problems with cocaine addiction, and probably other drugs). And he gave her — permanently gave her — our car because she had cracked hers up in an accident.

Never in my wildest dreams did I think all of this behavior was because of an incestuous relationship. But now, if it is true, it seems completely logical.

Is it any wonder, then, why he used his own daughter in a sexual way? Who knows what else went on in this family? I can't even think about it.

It's not an excuse for what he did to Sarah and me. Not in the least. He knew exactly what he was doing.

I didn't know any of that background information when we met with Dr. Chen, of course. And even if I had, would it have made any difference to the court and the authorities? My guess is, not at all.

A DAY IN COURT, PART 1

It is a warm day in L.A. when we arrive at the courthouse for an appearance related to the case. My husband Jim, my dad, my dad's wife, and I get there ahead of time so we won't be rushed. They always ask you to be outside the courtroom at 9 am, even though you never know exactly what time the judge will hear your case.

Mark, Lydia, Mark's mother and father, and Mark's sister Pam — the youngest of the three sisters, about two years older than Mark — are already there, too.

I remember being surprised at his sister's appearance; her multiple sclerosis had advanced quite a bit in the interim years since I'd seen her last. She used a cane and was thin and frail.

The halls outside family court have to be the most depressing place on earth. No one smiles. It's all very serious business, and since the cases are always so emotional, there is a heaviness in the air that makes you feel like you can't breathe without sobbing.

We avoid Mark and his family beforehand, not even looking at them directly. Eventually they move further down the hall, away from us.

Meanwhile, my family and I wait outside the courtroom, with our lawyer, until it is our turn. Three families go in before our case comes up. And each time, we notice the same thing happening.

After each ruling, the door bursts open, and the bailiff is escorting one of the two parties out the door. Invariably, the person being escorted is screaming, yelling, crying, looking like they are about to faint. Of the three people we witness, two are women and one is a man.

One of the women is so distraught, she almost appears to need a doctor.

I remember my dad saying, "What the heck is going on in there, anyway?" We are about to find out.

A DAY IN COURT, PART 2

So here we are, waiting our turn to see the judge. There are two main issues at hand:

1. Whether the judge was going to order all of us to see a second therapist/counselor, based on Dr. Chen's recommendations, and
2. I had asked for a raise in child support, as I had not requested one since our initial settlement in 1991, 9 years earlier.

I'll start with point #2. Our attorney, Peter, had done a very good job of presenting a case for a raise in child support. Under the law, I was entitled to request a raise every single year. I had never done so, mostly because I didn't want to confront Mark again. But since he had dragged us into the courtroom, it was a fair thing to address — especially since he had been paying the same amount for 9 years.

Mark was making a lot of money even when we were still married. His business had continued to improve, and he had quite a few material possessions to show for it: new cars, home remodeling, and the like. He could definitely afford to pay a couple hundred dollars more a month in child support (which, by the way, had nothing to do with the fact that I was remarried, under the law).

My lawyer stands up and asks the judge if he received the documents we submitted, requesting the raise in child support.

Judge: "Yes, I received them."

My lawyer: "Did you read them, your honor?"

Judge: "No, I didn't read them."

My lawyer stands there, his mouth gaping.

Judge: "Tell you what," he says, looking at me and then at Mark. "You two look like you make about the same amount of money, so I'm denying the raise in child support."

Bang of the gavel. My lawyer sits down and looks at me, mouthing, "What the F*&K just happened? I can't believe it!"

Now, to point #1, about all of us seeing a therapist/counselor.

After (supposedly) reading Dr. Chen's report, the judge orders that we see a counselor: Mark and Lydia, together; Sarah, on her own; and Jim and me, together. He orders that we all use the same counselor that is within 30 miles of where Jim, Sarah and I live (so that's good).

But then he drops a bombshell:

Judge: "And finally, I order that the defendant" — that

would be me — "pay all of the costs of the counseling on behalf of the plaintiff."

Bang of the gavel. Judge: "Next case."

I can't restrain myself.

I jump out of my seat and scream, "I have to PAY for his COUNSELING??! He sexually molested my child, and I have pay for his counseling??!!"

At that point, can you guess what happened?

Yes, the bailiff comes over to me, grabs me by the arm, and escorts me from the courtroom, as I keep on screaming.

After I am unceremoniously escorted out of the courtroom by the bailiff, I take off down the hall to try and compose myself. It doesn't work.

A couple of minutes later, I start running down the escalators (my family and attorney trailing several yards behind me). I scream the entire way down, so loudly that my voice is almost completely gone by the time I reach the courthouse lobby.

There, across the lobby, are Mark, Lydia, and Mark's family. With all the voice I have left, I yell at him:

"You think you can hide what you've done? I know EVERYTHING. EVERYTHING! You can lie to the court and fool everyone else. But NOT ME. You and I both know the truth. I know EVERYTHING!"

With that, I leave the courthouse and begin walking toward where we had parked the car, which was three or four blocks away.

After I walk about two blocks, my family finally catches up to me.

Once they reach me, I collapse onto the sidewalk: literally fall onto the asphalt, nearly hitting my head but managing to stop myself with my hands.

I immediately feel as if I were much too vulnerable — I don't want Mark to see me like that, so I beg my husband to get me up onto my feet as fast possible, which he does. He and my dad sort of drag me the two blocks to the car, with my dad's wife following just behind me, so in case Mark is walking somewhere nearby, he won't see the state I am in.

And what a state I was in.

All I could think of was: Here we are, all these years later, and once again, the court was ensuring that Sarah and I were paying for Mark's abuse — literally.

When someone files a lawsuit against you, no matter what the outcome is, you are screwed. There is no way to stop a lawsuit that someone has filed against you. The only way it stops is if the person who filed the lawsuit decides to end it.

Get the picture? As long as they have the money and resources to keep it going, they can. That's why you hear of lawsuits lasting years and years, because the person suing doesn't want to give up — and as long as they can pay and a judge agrees to hear the case, they don't have to stop.

Mark was paying his attorney "in kind," meaning, he was doing work for him instead of paying cash for his attorney's hourly fees.

As for us, we were paying our attorney the old-fashioned way: with every penny we had, credit cards, and money borrowed from family, too.

The lawsuit lasted nearly a year. I honestly have no idea

how much it cost, but it nearly put us into bankruptcy. At one point, I totaled up how much I, personally, had lost — money-wise — through the first divorce and custody battle and the second. The amount came to over $250,000.

For someone making a teacher's/writer's salary, $250,000 is a fortune. When I think of what we could have done with that money, like invest it and help pay for Sarah's education (including graduate school), it makes me sick.

One of Mark's tactics to hide his money revealed itself during this lawsuit. When I applied for a raise in child support, he claimed he had no cash assets. How did he do this?

His bank records showed he had one bank account that had $150,000 in cash in it. (I ask you, how does someone save that much IN CASH when they claim on their taxes that they're only making about $40,000 a year? I'll tell you how: they lie!)

But the day after he filed the lawsuit, he took that $150,000 and paid off the mortgage on his house.

Instead of, oh, giving some of it to Sarah to help pay for college, starting an investment fund for her, or giving her more in child support, he paid off his house and claimed he didn't have any money for her.

And he had no problem with jeopardizing her health and safety by nearly bankrupting her mother and stepfather.

Let's just say that on top of all the stress generated by the situation itself — that my daughter had been sexually abused by her father and his wife for her entire life — I also had to deal with the pain of financial disaster.

It was almost too much for me. When I had a month break from teaching at the university in December of 2000, I literally didn't leave the bedroom except to eat. It was difficult for me to face the reality of our lives.

But I had to. Because we now had to work with psychologist no. 2 — actually a marriage, family, child therapist named Bill. Bill would be the one to make the final recommendation to the court as to custody and visitation. So to say he was important would be putting it mildly.

BILL, THE COUNSELOR

Bill's office was just a half-hour drive from where we lived; Mark and Lydia had to drive nearly 3 hours to get there (which was fine by me!).

The office was located in a very plain building, in a parking lot across from a rather run-down department store. It wasn't a dangerous neighborhood, but it wasn't one that we frequented.

I believe the three of us went together for the first visit, although he may have set aside time to talk separately with Sarah, I can't quite recall.

What I do remember from that first meeting was trying to assess him and his abilities. Would he be able to see the truth clearly? Would he be able to see through Mark's lies?

Certainly he was very personable. His style was to listen and not say too much, at least at first. But he exuded a calm presence that set us at ease — well, as much as possible, anyway. The whole process was extremely stressful for all of us. There was so much at stake.

People may wonder, Wasn't she old enough at that point, 11 going on 12, to make up her own mind about where she wanted to spend time? If she didn't want to go to Mark's house anymore, what was the problem?

It just doesn't work that way.

Children have no rights. Abused children have no rights. All one has to do is read the paper or watch the news to see the truth of that statement.

Remember, family court's emphasis is on reunification, no matter what evidence appears in front of them suggesting that it's the wrong course.

For most of our appointments with Bill, I really couldn't get a good read on what he was thinking. Jim and I were honest with him; we told him everything, every detail we knew, about Sarah's and my experiences with Mark.

And I know Sarah was honest with Bill, too. I told her that this was a safe place for her to say anything she wanted to.

We saw Bill for several weeks — it might have even been 3 months or so. Most of what went on in those appointments is a blur to me now.

I do, however, remember the final two appointments with him.

TRYING TO BE NORMAL

I fake "normal." Because the fact is, I don't know what it means to have a normal life.

People may think that once you leave an abusive relationship, it's over. Move on. Let it go. All of that.

If you're reading this book and know someone who's been in my situation (or who has been through another type of serious trauma), I implore you to never say those words — move on, let go, it's in the past.

I am 50 years old now, and my daughter Sarah has graduated from college. Only now — only now — have I been able to start to deal with what has happened in my life. I've been seeing a counselor who specializes in domestic violence and sexual abuse, and I am starting to recognize how foggy and directionless my life has been, ever since the moment Mark raped me.

Because at that moment, my perspective on everything changed. I no longer felt a sense of possibility. I no longer thought of a future that could be interesting and filled with love, success, happiness.

Literally, all I wanted to do — this is the truth — is live to see Sarah turn 18. It's all I thought about. "If I can just live long enough to see Sarah turn 18, then I know she'll be free of Mark. She can do anything she wants."

I never thought about creating a future for myself, having a career, or anything like that. It was all about just staying alive long enough for Sarah to become a legal adult.

What I've learned is that this sense of living moment to moment, just getting through each day in one piece — even after the actual abuse has stopped — is "normal" for victims of domestic violence and sexual assault. It's how we see the world: minute by minute. We don't see the future, because we've been conditioned by abuse to react as if we wouldn't have one.

I'm trying to change that perspective now. I'm trying to be normal.

"NOTHING."

All five of us — Jim, me, Sarah, Lydia and Mark — saw Bill the counselor for several weeks, maybe months (I can't quite remember).

In April of 2001, things were winding down. We had just two sessions left, and then Bill would make his recommendation to the court as to whether Sarah had to see him any more.

The second-to-last session we had with Bill was memorable.

As always, Jim and I saw Bill separately from Sarah. At that particular session, we talked about quite a few things, one of which was my guilt over not being able to protect her during all the intervening years. Bill said to me, "When she was young, unless there was a mountain of physical evidence against Mark, there was nothing you could have done.

"Nothing."

It was only now, he explained, when Sarah was older, that the court would listen to her.

"Up until this age, the court would have paid no attention to what she had to say to me, or to you, or to anyone," he said. "The court doesn't listen to children."

He said all of this with a resignation and sadness that I hadn't seen in him before. It was the first time I really, truly felt he had been listening to everything we were telling him about Mark and Lydia. I started to feel some hope that maybe — dare I even think it? — things would go our way.

During that second-to-last session with Bill, even though I felt some glimmers of hope that he would see the truth and the court would listen, my fear was overwhelming.

At one point in the session, Bill looked me straight in the eye and asked me, "What do you want? What do you really want?"

I broke down. Completely broke down.

Through my hysterical sobbing, I screamed these words:

"I want him out of our lives! I WANT HIM OUT OF OUR LIVES!" With that, I fell to the floor of his office and literally wailed.

Jim and Bill let me express all of this emotion, then helped me back into the chair. Bill nodded at me. He looked me in the eye, and he nodded at me.

Did that mean he was going to try to help us get Mark out of our lives?

It was the final session, though, that was crucial. For Bill had determined that Sarah needed to confront Mark and Lydia directly. She had to tell them, in no uncertain terms, what they had done to her, how they had hurt her, and what she wanted to do about it.

How was she going to have the inner strength to do that? How would a 12-year-old girl have the intestinal fortitude to look her abusers — the people who had sexually molested her — in the eye and confront them with their crimes?

HELP FOR SARAH

In the weeks we were all seeing Bill, I was also taking Sarah to see another therapist for extra support. At these sessions, Sarah wanted me to stay in the room with her.

In the weeks leading up to the final session with Bill, when Sarah was to confront Mark and Lydia about the abuse, Annie worked with Sarah to figure out what she was going to say.

I worked with her, too. We would sit down every few days, and she would write some notes of things she had been thinking about. She used one of those composition books to help her keep everything straight.

While Sarah couldn't quite see the benefit of going to see Annie, I certainly did. Annie reinforced the fact that Sarah could confront them, that she had the power to do it, and that the environment Bill was providing was safe to do it.

Sarah was quite frightened. I think she knew it would ultimately be OK, but she was terrified.

But Annie would gently press her about her fears. Her favorite line was, "What's the worst that could happen?"

As strange as it sounds, that line had an impact on Sarah. She started to see that, in the confines of Bill's office, Mark would not be able to hurt her.

And maybe by telling him exactly what he did to her, Sarah could ensure that he would never hurt her again.

A DEPOSITION

I was remembering a deposition during this process in which I, myself, tried to confront Mark.

It was just like the first time, all these years before. Mark's lawyer asked me to describe what Sarah had told me — while Mark was sitting in the room, staring at me. As calmly as I could, which was nearly impossible, I told them everything. I began to tear up, and my throat started to close as I spoke about it.

And once again, Mark laughed.

What kind of man is that? I'm talking about abuse his daughter has suffered, that she says he has done to him, and he laughs.

At that, I lost control of my emotions. I stood up and the words just flooded out of me.

"Don't you understand what I'm trying to do here?" I said. "I'm trying to give you a way out. I'm trying to give you a chance to fess up to what happened, so that you can take responsibility for it, get help, and make amends. And then maybe, just maybe, you can have a relationship with your daughter. Don't you understand? DON'T YOU UNDERSTAND?"

At that point, the lawyers called a "recess" during the deposition.

I stepped into a nearby office that was empty, and started to cry. I was shaking uncontrollably.

The court reporter who had been taking everything down during the deposition saw me sitting there and came in.

There were tears in her eyes.

"I've been doing this a long time," she said to me. "And I'm so very, very sorry for what happened to you and your daughter. I've never seen someone act quite the way your ex-husband does. It's so terrible. He's so cruel. I'm truly sorry."

INTERMINABLE

Jim and I sat in the waiting room outside Bill's office for what seemed like hours, even though it was only 30 minutes.

Because Sarah was in Bill's office with Mark and Lydia, for the first time since all of this came out into the open.

Leading up to this day, Sarah had prepared herself to confront them both with what they had done to her. She had gotten support from another therapist and, of course, from Jim and me. The counselor, Bill, had also helped her.

I was nervous, uneasy, scared. I didn't know — couldn't know — what the effect of all of this might be on Sarah. Forget, for a moment, about the abuse all those years, and all the fear she had to live with: I knew what it was like to survive that and try to find my way. But actually confronting my abuser in person was something I knew nothing about.

Before she went in, I could see that she was steeling herself, trying not to cry. She hugged me, and she held her composition book close — the one with all her notes in it with what she was going to say.

The wait outside while she was talking to them was absolutely interminable. I was so tense I couldn't cry, or talk, or read, or anything. Jim tried to comfort me, but I asked him to please not say anything. I had to sit there in silence and stare at the door.

Before Sarah met with Mark and Lydia, she told me some — not all, as she wanted some privacy in this regard — of what she was going to say to them.

Part of it had to do with people changing their behavior.

At the end of her speech to them, she was planning to say that it didn't matter to her if he said he would change. She didn't believe him, and would never believe him.

"Because a leopard can't change his spots."

This revealed so much to me. It showed me that even though she was a child who, no doubt, still loved her father, she also knew him well. She held out no hope that he would ever change or even acknowledge what had happened or what he had done to her. Up until now, he had never, ever admitted the truth.

And of course, he had never apologized or even shown any concern for her well-being. Everything he had done — from filing the lawsuit in the first place, to denying he had any money in the bank — had shown his only concern was for himself.

While it saddened me, it also made me realize that she had reached a certain level of maturity. The idea of "wishful thinking" did not exist where Mark was concerned. Maybe somewhere, deep down, there was a glimmer of "I wish my dad would be a real dad to me." But it was slowly being snuffed out.

As terrible as this may sound, I was grateful for that. I didn't want her to live her life hoping for something that would never happen.

STILL CONTROLLING?

I have heard people say to victims of domestic violence, myself included, that they are still "allowing" the abuser to "control" them, long after they've left the relationship.

This thinking is so wrong, it's painful.

We take this view in our society, though. If the victim of a crime feels anything for a period of time afterward — lingering fear (or terror, even), grief, depression, what-have-you — we tell the victim, "You're letting the criminal control you. That means he still has power over you. So stop giving him that power!"

I used to think this way. And this way of thinking helped to deplete my self-esteem to the point where today, I barely have any left. It's another form of blaming the victim and then not understanding that there are real, palpable consequences of being the victim of a crime.

We don't want to see those long-term (or even short-term) consequences. They're ugly.

They make us uncomfortable.

So we try to force the victim to make it all nice for us. We ask her to forgive, so we don't have to deal with his behavior. We ask her to move on, so we can, too. We ask her to stop allowing him to control her life, so we can absolve ourselves of any societal responsibility for condoning his behavior in the first place. Next time you are about to suggest to someone who's been traumatized that they simply "let it go" and stop allowing the perpetrator to "control" their lives, please don't do it.

Instead, ask the victim what you can say or do to support them. And be willing to do it, whatever it is. Even if it means being uncomfortable.

ALL OF US TOGETHER

$\mathscr{L}$

Jim and I waited outside Bill's office while Sarah talked to Mark and Lydia, confronting them with what they did to her.

When Bill opened the door, Jim and I stood up quickly. I didn't hear anything from inside his office — no obvious crying — and Bill escorted us inside.

This was the first time Jim, Sarah and I had been in the same room with Mark and Lydia. I looked quickly at Sarah, who actually seemed quite composed, although it was clear she had shed a few tears. Lydia looked the most upset, as if she had been crying, and Mark was not showing a lot of emotion.

Jim and I sat with Sarah, and Bill spoke to all five of us. He didn't say much except to summarize what Sarah had told them, to make sure we all understood. And he ended with her comment, that even if Mark said he would change, she didn't believe him. "Because a leopard can't change his spots."

While Bill spoke, I watched Mark and Lydia to see how

they were reacting. Again, Lydia seemed very moved by everything. I really didn't — and don't — understand her. She was a party to the abuse and seemed perfectly willing to participate in everything. Unlike me, she didn't appear to be abused by Mark in any way. I realize women can hide things like that, because I certainly did, but I also knew what to look for — and I just didn't see any of the signs at all.

After he finished his summary, he asked Mark and Lydia to wait outside for a bit while he spoke to the three of us. My heart was racing. I just wanted all of this to be over with.

After Mark and Lydia left the room, Bill told Jim, Sarah and me that he was going to send his report and recommendation to the court the next day.

He had concluded that it was in Sarah's best interest that she not be forced, through court-ordered visitation, to see Mark anymore.

It was April of 2001. It was the first time since 1983, when I married Mark, that I finally felt free of him. My emotions ranged from disbelief — was this really happening? — to elation to fear — would he leave us alone now? — to relief.

We left Bill's office in a way that allowed us not to see Mark and Lydia as we exited the building. A couple of days later, our attorney called and said the judge had accepted Bill's recommendation.

None of us — not me, not Jim, not Sarah — have seen or spoken to Mark or Lydia since that day in Bill's office in April 2001.

CARDS & GRANDMOTHER

In the years that followed, Mark and Lydia sent a few cards for Sarah's birthday and at Christmas. But they quickly dwindled until they finally stopped showing up in the mailbox altogether. No gifts, no remembering her special days. No graduation present. No help with paying for college.

With the exception of one of Sarah's cousins (and the cousins' parents), no one in Mark's family stayed in touch with Sarah. Not her grandparents, not her other aunts or uncles or other cousins. No one. Mark had a fairly large family, but they cut her off just the way they had with me.

No one called. No one wrote.

She lost everyone. They all abandoned her.

We saw Mark's mother just once. Occasionally, Sarah's cousin would come visit us, so we'd meet her halfway when one of her parents drove her. On one of those trips, Sarah's grandmother — Mark's mother — had come along for the ride.

She was so happy to see Sarah, and Sarah was happy to see her. They hugged and cried and reminisced a little.

It had probably been at least two or three years since they had seen each other. I almost had the feeling, though, that she had sneaked out of the house. She didn't want to spend any extra time with Sarah — I had volunteered to take everyone out for a nice meal together — and only talked with us for about 15 or 20 minutes before getting back into the car to return to L.A.

That was the last time we saw her.

NORMAL?

As one might imagine, this story never really ends. Domestic violence, sexual assault and child sexual abuse have lifetime ramifications.

Most of the people in my life have no idea that I've been through all of this. Outwardly, I appear "normal." Many people I know — friends and colleagues who know nothing about this part of my life — have commented over the years about my ability to handle a lot of tasks with amazing calm. I suspect that ability comes, in part, from having a high degree of self-discipline and awareness. Mark "trained me," if you will, to be efficient while concealing my real feelings and hiding my weaknesses and fears.

Even today, my visage reveals little of what I've been through. I look young for my age; people are often genuinely surprised when I tell them I'm 50 and have a grown daughter.

That old saying of never really knowing what goes on behind closed doors? I am living proof of its truth.

Many women who have survived domestic violence bear the outward scars of abuse, but most of us do not. Domestic violence is truly a hidden societal malaise, with the added problem that both the perpetrators and their victims do not want it made known.

We have not had any contact at all with Mark or Lydia since their child support obligation ended when Sarah turned 18 – and even then, it was only in the form of the check in the mail. Neither one has admitted to the molestation. Neither one has reached out to Sarah or to us. We still have heard nothing from the rest of Mark's family, except for the cousin who has become Sarah's friend (the cousin's sister also has been in touch with her occasionally).

When Sarah turned 18, she made the decision to have Jim adopt her. It was a fairly easy process, but when we stood in that courtroom when they were legally made father and daughter — just the three of us, the judge and the court reporter — we cried. At least one time, a court appearance led to something good.

As of this moment, Sarah is living a good life. She graduated from a top university, has worked abroad and traveled, and is planning her future and setting professional and personal goals for herself.

Jim and I have been married for 14 years, but not altogether happily. The stress of the situation with Mark took a heavy toll on our relationship. And all of the associated problems I've had related to domestic violence have also played a significant role in our difficulties. We love each other and are trying to work through these problems to stay together.

I am seeing a counselor who specializes in working with victims of domestic violence and sexual assault. Only now can I see the incredible extent of the damage that was done to me by Mark.

One of the most shocking things has been the realization that I truly never envisioned a future for myself from the moment Mark first raped me. I've learned that this feeling of living moment-to-moment and just surviving is very common among people in my situation.

All I ever thought about was living long enough for Sarah to turn 18, when she would really be free of Mark.

As I've written before, I don't even know how to visualize myself beyond that goal. I don't know what I really want to do with my life. I know what my basic skills are, but the truth is, I'm not even sure what kind of person I am or what might make me happy. I don't know myself, because the self I was before, all those years ago before I knew Mark, is gone. She died in 1983, and I'm still grieving for her.

I look around at other people who haven't experienced trauma, and I wonder if they know what a gift it is to be able to actualize one's life, to make decisions and become something you actually want to be.

That's my task now: To find out who I am and what I want, to meet and accept the self that I am now.

I just hope I have some time left, at 50, to make something of my life. Some days I think I can. Most days, though, I feel empty and blank, a shell of a person who has never really lived a day in her adult life. It's been an existence, nothing more: a pretense of normal, without a connection to what "normal" even means.

Over time, the title of this book has taken on new meaning for me. When I look in the mirror, often that's all I see: just a woman. Someone who exists inside a female body, and that's all.

I could lie and say that I honestly believe I can create a future for myself, that I can construct some reasonable semblance of a person out of the woman in the mirror. But it's not the truth, at least not today.

Maybe tomorrow I will feel differently.

* * *

THIS CONCLUDES THE ORIGINAL MEMOIR. PLEASE READ THE EPILOGUE FOR THE REST OF THE STORY …

EPILOGUE

THE HAPPY ENDING STARTS HERE

I never thought I'd be able to write a happy ending to the story of my life.

Now granted, my life isn't over just yet (thank goodness!). As I'm writing this epilogue, it is 2017. I'm about to turn 56 years old and am in excellent health.

But with what I know today, I can say with absolute certainty that there is zero chance that I'll ever experience the unhappiness, desperation, stress and despair that I felt for so many years.

No more post-traumatic stress disorder.

No more effects of trauma.

I'm at peace.

I'm happy.

Joyful.

Even giddy sometimes.

And those feelings aren't going anywhere.

Gosh, did I really say that — and mean it?
Yes.

It sounds a bit crazy, honestly. Especially when I read what I wrote in this memoir.

So what happened? How did I go from the depths of PTSD to where I am now?

That's what I'll share with you in this epilogue.

IN THE FALL OF 2013, ABOUT 18 MONTHS AFTER WRITING AND SELF PUBLISHING THE ORIGINAL EDITION OF THIS BOOK, I WAS NOT DOING WELL.

I was filled with feelings of dread, anxiety and worry that wouldn't go away no matter what I did. I tried meditating, walking, listening to music, reading, writing, going to the movies, knitting, something called "tapping" (Emotional Freedom Technique) and all kinds of other techniques. I saw my most recent therapist a couple more times, too.

Nothing helped.

I WAS DESPERATE.

I wanted the PTSD gone. For good.

However, I didn't think it was possible. In fact, I was sure that PTSD was a permanent condition: an incurable mental illness. That's what I had been told for decades, and certainly my symptoms suggested that it was true.

At the time — as evidenced by the previous chapters in this book — I believed that I was broken. No way to "fix" me.

BY ALL ACCOUNTS, I SHOULD HAVE BEEN FEELING GOOD.

When I released the original edition of this book, I had just completed an intensive 16-month psychotherapy process. My second marriage, to Jim, was improving. Jim and I had been having trouble in our relationship for a long time, but we had begun resolving many of our problems, and things were looking up.

But instead of feeling happy, I noticed that my symptoms of PTSD were cropping up all the time and all over the place: on the subway, at home, at work, in my relationships, and as I walked the streets of New York City, where I was living at the time.

And wow, was I mad about that!

I thought, "I have done all this work in the therapist's office. I have spent countless hours learning coping techniques, writing in my journal and all the rest. I've seen so many mental health professionals, more than I can count, and still, I have no relief. What else am I supposed to do?"

I concluded that, sure enough, I really was broken — never to be whole again. Never to be the person I was before my ex-husband began abusing me and, later, my daughter.

I fell into a deeper state of grief.

I WAS INCREDIBLY FRUSTRATED, BECAUSE WHAT I WANTED FROM LIFE DIDN'T SEEM THAT FAR FETCHED.

All I wanted was to feel at peace.

I'd look at people — friends, family members, strangers —

who hadn't been through something traumatic, and I was so jealous I could barely stand it. I wanted what they had. I'd watch them smile and laugh without worry, and I'd see them pursuing their dreams and goals fearlessly, and my insides would seethe with anger.

Sometimes the envy was so overpowering, I wanted to scream, "Why did this have to happen to me, and to my child? Why can't I turn back the clock and make a different decision, so I can just be happy?"

I was in emotional agony.

AT THE END OF 2013, I MADE A DECISION THAT I THOUGHT WOULD LEAD TO MORE HAPPINESS IN MY LIFE.

In truth, it felt more like grasping at the end of a frayed rope.

What did I do? I decided to become a life coach.

Yes, I know. It sounds completely nutty to me now, considering the state of mind I was in. But I didn't think I could get any better, so what the heck? I knew I had the skills to coach people because I had been a teacher for several years. I also believed that my personal experiences with domestic violence could be helpful to someone.

Simply put, I wanted to do something meaningful with my life.

So I enrolled in a coach-training program.

In the beginning, everything seemed fine. But a few weeks into the training, I knew that something was missing in what I was learning. The training itself seemed like there was a hole in the middle of it, and I couldn't figure out exactly what was wrong.

One day, on my lunch break from my day job, I sat down next to a tree in Central Park. I set up my iPhone, and I recorded a video to post on my coaching website. In that video, I talked a bit about my experience with domestic violence, and I remember stating that I finally realized that being happy was a choice.

Even while I was saying those words, I knew they were a lie. I shed tears while I was talking, but not because I was talking about my violent first marriage. It was because I knew I wasn't telling the truth.

I posted the video, anyway.

At the time, I didn't know what else to believe. The psychotherapy process seemed to tell me the same thing, as did the entire self-development world and, certainly, the coach-training program I was in. The message was always something like this: "Mary, you can be happy whenever you want to. You just have to change your thinking to be more positive, more present, more accepting of your life, and then you can choose to be happy."

Ugh!

I didn't want to accept my life as it was. No way!

Plus, over the years I had tried and tried, but I couldn't choose, change or create any of my thoughts, let alone happy ones. I mean, who *wouldn't* do that if they could? And as a coach, I certainly didn't want to try to make other people do something that wouldn't work. What a waste of time!

By mid-2014, I was frustrated, sad and worn out.

But something inside kept nagging at me, saying, "There must be an answer, Mary. Don't give up."

Despite everything, hope stayed alive within me.

I soon discovered why …

A CHANCE ENCOUNTER WITH A BOOK

One day in mid-2014, I was surfing the web when I ran across a video of someone talking about a book they had read and the impact it had made on their life.

Now normally, I don't watch these kinds of videos. This time, though, something drew me in. Perhaps it was the speaker's enthusiasm, I don't know. But after watching the video for the full 45 minutes and not really "getting" what the person was saying, I was still intrigued. I went onto Amazon and bought the paperback, the Kindle version and the Audible recording of *The Inside-Out Revolution*, by Michael Neill.

To say I was skeptical would be an understatement. After all, the subtitle of the book was, "All you need to know to change your life forever."

I thought to myself, "What an arrogant thing to say! Who is this Michael Neill, anyway? He must have a huge ego to think he knows what would change *my* life."

Even so, I started reading — or rather listening to — the

book. I listened to it on my subway commute to work, during breaks and on my lunch hour. When I finished it the first time through, I remember thinking, "What is he talking about? I don't understand."

Just as before, though, hope prodded me to keep going.

So I listened to the book again. Every day, I'd get home from work and look through the paperback and Kindle versions, too, trying to decipher what this author was saying.

I KNEW THIS: SOMETHING IN THE BOOK WAS DIFFERENT, VERY DIFFERENT, FROM ANYTHING I HAD HEARD BEFORE.

One day, I went out for my usual lunchtime walk and — as had become my habit — I listened to the book. About thirty minutes into my walk, I stopped at an island in the middle of a big intersection near Lincoln Center and sat down on one of the benches there. The weather had begun to get warmer and more humid, and there were pink and purple impatiens planted in big pots. The flowers looked really beautiful to me, their colors glowing in the bright sunlight.

I heard the Michael Neill's voice in my headphones, and with the suddenness of a lightning bolt, something changed — almost like I'd woken up from a bad dream and realized I was safe.

A flood of joy, peace, success, security, fulfillment and love washed over me. Sitting on that stupid little bench in the middle of gigantic New York City, I cried the happiest tears I had ever had.

In that instant — it really was instantaneous — my whole world, my whole life, changed.

I know this might sound unbelievable, but it's true.

What I heard wasn't religion, philosophy or even spirituality, as I'd been exposed to it. Been there, done that.

No, this was different. Big. The biggest.

I went back to my office in a delightful haze, and I emailed the life coach training program and told them that I was quitting …

THE TRUTH

What happened next is pretty funny when I look back on it. After quitting the coach training, I bought copies of Michael Neill's book and gave it to several key people in my life. I also talked about the book and its message with anyone who would listen to me.

I couldn't help myself. *I finally knew the truth.* Two truths, actually, occurred to me on that bench on the middle of Broadway:

1) I wasn't ill or broken, and I never had been (*yowza!*).

2) I had been creating my own suffering, and it was actually easy — yes, easy — to stop doing that.

LET'S DISCUSS THE FIRST TRUTH: I AM NOT BROKEN. AND NEITHER ARE YOU.

No matter what had happened to me in the past, no matter

what might happen to me in the future, I could never, ever be broken, harmed, chipped — nothing.

Just like every other human being, I am unbreakable. Shatterproof. Even when I die, I will still be whole.

How do I know? Because I saw with certainty that I'm not the thoughts that go through my head, nor am I this body I'm inhabiting. It's like there is a "little Mary," the one who is comprised of this body, listening to thoughts and eating and drinking and all of that stuff; and there's also "Big Mary," which cannot be contained by thoughts or by this human form.

I — the real me — am not the "little Mary" but the "Big Mary": an innately whole, innately healthy being that cannot be touched, harmed or contained by anything or anyone.

In short, there was nothing wrong with me. I had never been sick at all.

I remember thinking to myself, "Why didn't anyone tell me this before?"

If even one, just one, of the mental health professionals I had spoken to had seen me as healthy and whole, and not as someone with a mental illness, that would have made all the difference to me.

But that's not what happened. Instead, they all sat across from me and viewed me as "ill," as someone who needed to learn how to "cope," when actually, *I was 100 percent fine the whole time!*

I'll come back to this idea in a moment, but let's move on, for now.

THE SECOND TRUTH IS THAT THOUGHTS CREATE OUR MOMENT-TO-MOMENT EXPERIENCE AND OUR FEELINGS, BUT WE DON'T HAVE TO DO ANYTHING ABOUT THEM.

I always knew that the thoughts swirling through my head had something to do with my suffering from PTSD. I just didn't understand the role of thoughts, overall.

After reading *The Inside-Out Revolution*, I caught a glimpse of something brand new and realized that I had been unwittingly creating my own suffering.

Before coming to this new understanding of myself, I believed my ex-husband was responsible for my suffering. After all, he had harmed my daughter, he had harmed me, and he had done irreparable damage to my life.

With a new view on things, I saw that a) he hadn't harmed me at all (see the first truth, above), and b) the only thing I was actually experiencing were the thoughts going through my mind. I was giving weight to these thoughts, believing them, seeing them as truth — when in fact, they weren't true at all.

Not only that, nothing on the "outside" was creating any feelings in me, either. Only thoughts can do that. It's impossible for feelings to be transmitted from a person or thing "out there" and into us (unless we're waving a magic wand, like Harry Potter!).

Wait, what was that?

I'll say it again. *Nothing, and no one, on the "outside" creates our feelings. Only thoughts do that.*

Being slightly (OK, more than slightly) skeptical, I decided to test this out.

For several weeks, I ran experiments. Was something or someone on the "outside" causing a feeling in me? Or was it really my thinking doing that?

For instance, one day I'd be sitting on the subway and have no symptoms of PTSD. The next day — same conditions — I'd be riding the subway and feel so anxious, I'd want to run screaming from the car every time the doors opened.

How was that possible?

On the first day, my thoughts weren't stressful. On day two, my thoughts were stressful, I was listening to them — and I was agreeing with them!

The final proof was seeing that obviously, my ex-husband was nowhere to be found on the subway, so where was the suffering originating? It certainly couldn't be coming from him, nor was it coming from the people sitting near me reading their books and playing games on their iPhones.

Indeed, my suffering was coming from the thoughts I was listening to.

HERE'S THE KICKER: I DISCOVERED THAT I HAD THE OPTION TO IGNORE MY THOUGHTS. I DIDN'T HAVE TO "MANAGE" THEM (BECAUSE I CAN'T, AND NEITHER CAN YOU).

During my experiments, I simply sat with the feeling of anxiety and did nothing. Those thoughts and feelings came and went as they pleased. Instead of trying to manage my thoughts — which I have concluded is impossible — I just ignored them.

I felt whatever feeling I had and didn't worry about it. I knew the first truth, which is that nothing could possibly break me, so I was no longer afraid of my feelings.

I'll say that again: *I was no longer afraid of my feelings.*

I didn't care what they were because they were simply mirroring thoughts I was having right then, and nothing more.

Our feelings don't signify anything; they are merely a reflection of whatever thoughts are floating through our head at any given moment.

My whole adult life, before seeing this new view on my experience, every time I had a PTSD-type symptom I tensed with worry and anxiety. I thought it meant something significant, like my life was crap, my mental health was crap, like everything was crap.

But with a new understanding, if I had a symptom — like anxiety or whatever — I didn't worry at all. It was a passing thought/feeling.

I realized, *So what?* Everyone has thoughts. Everyone has feelings that result from thoughts. It's how human beings operate.

As a result, thoughts and feelings no longer looked like a big deal. They looked normal and, ultimately, kind of neutral.

Within just six weeks of realizing these two truths I've been talking about, and simply doing nothing when I felt uncomfortable, my PTSD symptoms faded away.

They have never returned.

This, after having seen more than 25 (mostly) well-meaning mental health professionals, and after having tried every technique and tool imaginable.

Why does doing nothing actually help?

Doing nothing works because of the first truth: that you and I are born with innate health and well-being, and it's running beneath the surface of our lives 24/7. It's our natural set point, if you will — like the place a pendulum comes to rest when it stops swinging back and forth between emotions, which happens much more effortlessly when we don't worry about the swings.

OVER TIME, I HAVE COME TO SEE THOUGHTS AS BEAUTIFUL GIFTS.

Thoughts allow us to have this amazing and powerful "human being experience": emotional highs, lows and everything in between.

The difference now is that I know our thoughts don't mean anything. Instead of paying attention to them all day or worrying about them, we can listen to something else — to what is beyond our thoughts, to what is, essentially, the source of our thoughts. What is that? It is who we really are.

WE ARE NOT OUR THOUGHTS. WE ARE SO MUCH MORE.

A few months after this life-changing discovery, something happened that was a true turning point — and one that I never expected …

A TURNING POINT

One of the emotions that plagued me all those years was hatred.

I didn't look hateful on the outside, but I carried a whole big pile of hatred around with me every day. No matter how I tried, I could not understand why my ex-husband did what he did. Over and over again, I'd ask myself that nagging question: *Why?*

I held Mark in complete contempt. I hated him.

As I wrote in the original book, I was never going to forgive Mark for what he had done. To me, his actions were unforgivable.

One evening, several months after first reading *The Inside-Out Revolution* and having that life-changing moment on the bench on Broadway, I had a major turning point while waiting for the subway at 79th Street.

I had just finished my workout at the gym and was going home. The subway station was nearly deserted, so I was standing alone on the platform, leaning against one of the posts and eating a nutrition bar (chocolate, my favorite).

OUT OF NOWHERE, I HAD A NEW THOUGHT.

Mark and I were the same.

Wow.

Mark and I were the same.

Mark had certain thoughts that he was listening to and believing, and then acting upon them — just as I did.

His thoughts had convinced him that in order to feel secure, he had to lash out. He also saw other people as the cause of his suffering. To remedy that, he tried to control them.

My thoughts had convinced me that I was broken inside, so I suffered. I, too, tried to control my environment and sometimes my thoughts in order to feel better, not realizing that my environment had nothing to do with my feelings and that I didn't have to control my thoughts.

AND THEN, I HAD ANOTHER NEW THOUGHT.

Mark and I were also the same because both of us were innately whole and healthy. No matter how he had behaved, that behavior was reflecting momentary thinking that he was reacting to, *not who he was as a human being.*

Double wow.

In a flash, I saw Mark as someone who was suffering deeply because he hadn't seen what I had seen.

Let me be clear: I wasn't excusing his behavior, and I would never do that. Do I wish it hadn't happened? Of course. More than anything, I wish my daughter had been spared everything she went through.

BUT FINALLY, I HAD THE ANSWER TO MY NAGGING QUESTION, "WHY?"

Mark was living with a misunderstanding of who he actually was. If he had known that security, for example, was innate, he would have felt no need to hurt people. If he had known that his feelings came from momentary thoughts, he wouldn't have tried to control other people — because people cannot create feelings in us. Only thoughts do that. And he could have simply waited for a new and better thought to come into his mind, instead of reacting.

When the subway train arrived, I was crying uncontrollably. I got into the car and found a seat. A woman sitting next to me handed me a tissue and asked if I was all right. I nodded *Yes*, wishing I could tell her just how all right I actually was.

My anger, my contempt, my hatred toward Mark … it was all gone, never to return.

In the past, I didn't know what I would do if I ever saw Mark again. I feared I might punch him.

If I saw Mark today, I would probably hug him.

MOTHERHOOD, REBORN

In re-reading this memoir, I was touched by the immense grief I experienced related to motherhood. According to the final therapist I saw, because of all the trauma I had been through I simply couldn't be the mother to Sarah that I would have been otherwise.

To say that that news was crushing would be an understatement.

Today, all that has changed. Happily, the therapist was wrong. Innocently wrong, but still wrong.

I CAN SEE QUITE CLEARLY THAT I WAS — AND STILL AM — THE MOTHER I HAD ALWAYS WANTED TO BE.

In motherhood, as in many areas of my life, the innate well-being that I've been talking about in this epilogue had fully risen to the surface. The ease with which I raised Sarah, and the enduring love between us, is evidence of this truth.

A while back, Sarah was staying with her stepdad Jim and me in New York City, and she fell ill with a physical symptom that I knew could be potentially fatal. We rushed her to the emergency room, and without waiting a moment, we were whisked inside, and a doctor examined her.

He told us what we already knew: that it could be nothing, or it could be something deadly.

At one point, she needed to get a scan of her head, so as she was wheeled on the gurney into the waiting area for radiology, I went with her.

I sat down in a chair next to the gurney, and I was crying. So was she. We were afraid, and we knew that the results of the scan would determine whether she would live … or not. It was that serious.

We looked into each other's eyes, and in those few moments, we had the most beautiful conversation I can ever remember us having. It almost seemed like we weren't actually speaking out loud, and the sensation was of the two of us as one living, breathing being — no distance between us at all.

The hospital faded into the background, as did our fears. Although the fearful thinking was still present, it wasn't having any effect on us. We talked about some wonderful times we'd shared, like going to Disneyland many times over the years.

And finally, she said, "It's always been you and me, Mommy."

Fortunately, the tests were negative. But I will never forget that conversation — proof that nothing, not even severe violence or all the stressful thinking I had been listening to all those years, could diminish the one thing I had always wanted in life: to be a good mom.

THE HAPPY ENDING CONTINUES

After informally sharing what I had discovered for a couple of years, in early 2016 I made the decision to leave my previous career in communications and become a professional coach: helping people live happier, less stressful and more successful lives. In addition to coaching people, I began writing and self publishing short books that illustrate, in the best way that I can, these two truths: that we cannot ever be broken, and that momentary, transient thinking (normal and nothing to worry about) is creating our experience as human beings but is not who we really are.

In early 2016, I met author and coach Michael Neill in person when he came to New York City to give a talk. By that time, I had taken a couple of his online group programs, so he knew my name. As I walked up to him, he opened his arms and said, "Is this THE Mary Schiller?" We hugged each other, and I thanked him for changing my life.

Since then, I've been fortunate to have several people tell

me the same thing after reading my books, which has been more rewarding than I could have ever dreamed.

Later in 2016, Michael interviewed me on his Hay House Radio program. I shared a bit about my experience with domestic violence and recovery and talked about one of my books. It was a magical moment for me.

There have been many magical moments since 2014 — too many to count.

As I'm writing this section of the book, I am now living in Paris, France — the realization of a dream I've had since I was 19 years old. I'm writing more books, coaching people, spending time with Jim and Sarah and, with the publication of this book using my real name, embarking on a whole new journey.

In short, my experience of life has changed completely. Looking back on my life up until now, everything has a subtle but unmistakable sheen to it. No more regret, no more wishing I had made different choices.

Gone are the PTSD symptoms, the anger, the grief, the hatred. In their place is a deep sense of peace that I never believed was possible for me.

My life — all of it, from my very first memory until now — looks beautiful to me.

Not only that, but I've seen that I have permission to do what I want to do with this life of mine, and I'm having so much fun every day doing only things I enjoy: writing, coaching amazing people, making new friends and staying close to my "forever friends," spending time with my husband

and daughter, exploring Paris ... it's everything I could have ever wanted.

Little did I know that the peace I was searching for wasn't just within me.

It IS me.

And it is you, too.

It is all of us.

WHAT TO DO NEXT

If you'd like to learn more about what has changed my life and the lives of thousands of other people, here are some suggestions:

- Read my books *The Joy Formula: The simple equation that will change your life*; and *Mind Yoga: The simple solution to stress that you've never heard before (no stretchy pants required)*. I wrote those two short books as easy-to-understand introductions to what I've shared with you in this epilogue.
- Read Michael Neill's *The Inside-Out Revolution: The only thing you need to know to change your life forever*. I always recommend this book, and it's my favorite of his offerings.
- Enroll in my free course, "Unleash Your Courage." Discover how simple — and fun — it is to tap into the courage that is innately yours. Visit the

website www.unleashyourcouragenow.com to sign up. Again, the class is free.
- Get in touch with me at mary@maryschiller.com. I'd love to hear from you. I also have several free resources — like interviews and such — at www.maryschiller.com.

IF THIS BOOK HAS BEEN HELPFUL TO YOU, PLEASE WRITE A REVIEW ON THE WEBSITE WHERE YOU PURCHASED IT.

It's not just for me, although of course I appreciate it. Your review will increase the book's ranking, so people searching for a book related to domestic violence and PTSD will be able to find it. So you'll be helping even more people along with me! Thank you so much.

I always say that if this new understanding can help me, it can help anyone.

THERE IS HOPE. THERE IS AN ANSWER.

I'm living proof.
Much love to you,
Mary

ABOUT THE AUTHOR

Mary Schiller is an author and coach who helps people experience less stress and more joy and success in their lives.

Before she began her career as an author and coach, Mary taught college students how to write the perfect essay and worked in communications for an Ivy League university. She holds advanced degrees in English and in education.

A native Californian, Mary is passionate about classical music (Beethoven is unmatched), art, photography and knitting. She's married and has a grown daughter plus two adorable cats and currently lives in Paris, France.

Mary is available to give talks about her experience with domestic violence and recovery to your group, organization or company. Please connect with Mary to learn more.

Enroll in the free course, "Unleash Your Courage." Visit www.unleashyourcouragenow.com.

Get in touch:
www.maryschiller.com
mary@maryschiller.com

ALSO BY MARY SCHILLER

The Joy Formula: The simple equation that will change your life

Mind Yoga: The simple solution to stress that you've never heard before (no stretchy pants required)

A-ha! How to solve any problem in record time

To Love is to Listen: Transform your relationships & your life with a powerful new way to listen

You Have Permission: How to stop doing stuff you don't want to do and start doing stuff you do want to do

How to Be Happy When You're Broke

How to Be Happy in the Age of Trump

Printed in Great Britain
by Amazon